PARAMEDICAL
PATHOLOGY

PARAMEDICAL PATHOLOGY

Fundamentals of Pathology for the Allied Medical Occupations

By

ALVIN F. GARDNER, Ph.D (Pathology)

Bureau of Drugs, Food and Drug Administration
Department of Health, Education and Welfare
Washington, D. C.
Formerly Associate Professor of Pathology
School of Dentistry and Graduate School
University of Maryland, Baltimore, Maryland
Formerly Consultant in Pathology
U. S. Public Health Service and
Veteran's Administration
Baltimore, Maryland

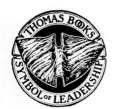

CHARLES C THOMAS · PUBLISHER
Springfield · Illinois · U.S.A.

Published and Distributed Throughout the World by

CHARLES C THOMAS • PUBLISHER

Bannerstone House

301-327 East Lawrence Avenue, Springfield, Illinois, U.S.A.

Natchez Plantation House

735 North Atlantic Boulevard, Fort Lauderdale, Florida, U.S.A.

© *1972 by* CHARLES C THOMAS • PUBLISHER

ISBN 0–398–02289–5

Library of Congress Catalog Card Number: 70–184596

This book was written by Dr. Gardner in his private capacity. No official
support or endorsement by the Department of Health, Education and
Welfare is intended or should be inferred.

Printed in the United States of America

K-8

To my wife

ESTHER VITA

In appreciation of her sympathetic assistance and devotion. Without her encouragement this book would not have been written.

PREFACE

The allied medical occupations were relatively unknown occupations a few decades ago. Numerous colleges and hospitals have recently entered into the allied medical training fields in the form of a major endeavor by offering numerous allied medical courses. The education of allied medical personnel is backed by federal optimism and federal funds. Many medical educators and medical practitioners believe, and rightly so, that tremendous expansion will occur in the nation's leading training centers for allied medical careers. Students will be attending schools of allied medical occupations on multimillion-dollar campuses adjacent to hospitals throughout the United States and Canada.

The need for trained allied medical personnel will continue to stay well ahead of the available personnel for decades to come. Allied medical occupations are increasing in importance and a fundamental knowledge of general pathology is essential to meet the needs of the present day and future members of these various occupations. With the growing number and complexity of courses for allied health personnel constantly increasing and changing, pathology becomes the basis and most vital background upon which all advanced and future courses can be based.

The current allied medical occupations encompass the following fifteen occupations: registered nurse, certified laboratory assistant, cytotechnologist, inhalation therapy technician, medical assistant, medical record librarian, medical record technician, medical technologist, nuclear medicine technician, occupational therapist, physical therapist, radiation therapy technologist, radiologic technologist, orthopedic assistant, and histologic technician.

The allied health graduates from the above allied health occupations, which should number 100,000 annually in the next decade, can achieve their major task only if they complete a course in the fundamentals of general pathology during their allied health curriculum. This book has been prepared especially for the student and graduate of allied health occupations and is applicable to the personnel of all the categories enumerated above.

This treatise represents a presentation of the fundamentals of general pathology prepared for the allied medical occupations. This treatise takes into account the experiences that well prepared students and members of these numerous occupations have had in dealing with the basic concepts of the biomedical sciences. It is therefore assumed that the personnel using this book have the background, capacity and desire to obtain a considerable understanding of pathologic processes. In order to help make this understanding possible, basic concepts and pathologic terms are presented in the first half of this book.

Pathology is an exciting, rapidly changing, and vital area of the biological and medical sciences which provides an excellent and important background for all students and members of the allied health occupations. The study of pathology presents limitless possibilities to continue with advanced and post-graduate studies in the various allied medical occupations. It is important that a book of this type be made available to the members of these fields so that the important features of pathology can be stressed and other areas reduced to a minimum. Only in this manner will the members of the allied health occupations be able to obtain a greater appreciation of human disease processes. For instance, pathology teaches the allied medical personnel that good hygiene is the best safeguard to their health. The breath expelled by a tuberculous patient during coughing contains a fine spray of droplets which may be laden with tubercle bacilli. The allied health personnel should try to avoid inhaling it, and should periodically have a chest x-ray.

The members of the allied health occupations are engaging in an art based upon fundamental pathologic knowledge and clinical practice. A sound foundation in human pathologic processes is vital in order to carry out clinical procedures with meticulous care. Logical simplicity has been considered of utmost importance in order to encourage the allied health personnel to enlarge their knowledge of pathology.

It is the author's hope that this book will enhance the current and future potentials of all allied health occupations by providing the members of the allied health teams with the basic science fundamentals of pathology. Only with this knowledge of pathology can the allied health occupations equip their present and future students for successful clinical practices.

ALVIN F. GARDNER

CONTENTS

PARAMEDICAL
PATHOLOGY

Chapter 1

INTRODUCTION TO THE STUDY OF
PATHOLOGY FOR
THE ALLIED MEDICAL OCCUPATIONS

Pathology is an applied science which is broader in scope than the basic allied medical sciences. Pathology is distinctive because it is a medical science and a correlated clinical field of medicine. Pathology is readily correlated with all of the basic medical sciences and with therapeutics. It represents the bridge between the basic sciences and the clinical and therapeutic aspects of medicine. The word *pathology* is derived from *pathos,* meaning disease, and *logos,* meaning discourse. The morphologic alteration is now considered to be of equal importance with alterations in tissue physiology, biochemistry and histochemistry. Pathology is many sciences correlated into one field. In medicine, pathology is a correlated medical science and is composed of human biology as well as therapeutics.

FUNDAMENTAL DEFINITIONS IN THE STUDY OF PATHOLOGY

The term *disease* means that there is a disturbance in the function, morphology and biochemistry of the cell, tissue or organ. *Lesions* are the clinical manifestations of disease which are utilized to identify the disease process. *Etiology* is the study of the causation of disease. *Pathogenesis* is the method of development of a pathologic process from inception to the termination of a disease. *Life history* of a disease is the most commonly expected course which a disease follows from inception to termination without alterations due to therapeutics. *Diagnosis* is the recognition of a specific pathologic process arrived at by subjective and clinical manifestations. *Prognosis* is the forecasting of how the specific pathologic process will terminate based on the life history of the disease plus the individual's ability to adequately respond to therapeutics. *Pathognomonic* is the specific characteristic (s) indicative of a particular disease.

ETIOLOGY OF SYSTEMIC DISEASES

Diseases should be viewed as having a complex etiology. The causes of disease may be *intrinsic* or *extrinsic.* Extrinsic nonliving causes include force, sound, light, electricity, irradiation, chemicals, heat, cold and atmospheric pressure. Extrinsic living factors include bacteria, fungi, viruses, rickettsia, spirochetes, protozoa and metazoa. Intrinsic causes of disease are due to congenital, inherited, metabolic, hormonal and neurogenic factors.

The cause of disease may be classified as *exciting* in nature. A microorganism is the exciting factor in an infection. *Precipitating* causes of disease are those secondary factors which support the action of the exciting causes. *Predisposing* causes are those factors which prepare for or favor the development of disease, i.e. disturbance of nutrition, racial factors and smoking.

CLASSIFICATION OF SYSTEMIC DISEASES

Congenital diseases are faults in intrauterine development which are present at birth. Not all congenital diseases are inherited, some are acquired *in utero* while others are of unknown etiology.

Inherited diseases are due to the transmission of inherent characteristics in one or both parents from one generation to another. These diseases may be present at birth and are thus congenital and hereditary. When they appear after birth they are inherited but not congenital.

Traumatic diseases are the result of direct physical forces or chemical injury resulting in disturbances in the affected tissues.

Infectious and granulomatous diseases are the result of living extrinsic bacteria, viruses, parasites, fungi and worms invading the human body.

Allergic diseases are provoked in an individual hypersensitive to a particular substance or group of substances.

Degenerative diseases are the result of retrograde changes in cells and premature aging of tissues.

Neoplastic diseases are the result of an uncontrolled new growth of cells which proliferates rapidly, invades adjacent tissue and spreads to distant sites.

Nutritional diseases are due to an inadequate intake of essential body nutrients and to an imbalance or excessive intake of nutrients.

Metabolic diseases are the result of a disturbance in the normal function of organs or systems, such as endocrine imbalances or disturbances in intrinsic metabolic functions.

GENERAL ADAPTATION SYNDROME IN SYSTEMIC DISEASES

Isolated destruction of individual cell groups results in an interaction between damage, and the defense on the part of the remaining cells is defined as *stress* by Selye.* Specific effects are characteristic of one or a few pathogens—for instance, Koplik spots in the oral mucosa are characteristic of measles. Other pathogens are nonspecific. Nonspecific pathogens may be local or systemic. Inflammation is an example of a local effect of a nonspecific pathogen. The systemic nonspecific effects of pathogens refer to the *General Adaptation Syndrome*. A pathogen may produce a circumscribed inflammation which is a local nonspecific change. In addition, systemic manifestations occur with mild general adaptation syndrome changes, i.e. slight

* Selye, H.: Stress—The physiology and pathology of exposure to stress. *Acta* (Montreal), 1950. Seyle, H.: The general adaptation syndrome as a basis for unified theory of medicine. *Oral Surg, 5:* 408, 1952.

ACTH discharge will be superimposed upon the local nonspecific changes. Extensive traumatic injuries produce predominantly nonspecific effects, i.e. extreme inflammation with intense ACTH discharge.

The clinical manifestations of most systemic diseases will represent a mixture of specific and nonspecific stress effects. The manifestations of systemic diseases are the result of the interactions between the nonspecific and specific stress. All pathogens act directly or indirectly upon cells. The most nonspecific type of reaction that any pathogen can elicit is necrosis. The most highly specific type of reaction is abnormal mitosis. Therefore, the general adaptation syndrome states that a specific reaction could be due to stress if the pathogen be directed selectively upon certain structures. Before the disease spreads from the cell to the body as a whole, it goes through a clearly defined intermediate step, that of limitation of further spread by defense mechanisms in the local area. It has become increasingly more evident that in addition to the local responses, the entire body participates in all disease processes whether local or systemic. The systemic reaction is possible only through the humoral and nervous system.

Chapter 2

FORMS OF TISSUE INJURY—CELL DEGENERATION AND NECROSIS

CELLULAR DEGENERATIVE PROCESSES AND INFILTRATIONS

Disturbances of Intracellular Proteins

Hypoproteinemia. The circulation is a mobile fluid dependent on the hydrostatic and osmotic pressure of the plasma proteins. The balance between the fluid within the blood vessels and the extravascular fluid depends upon maintaining the level of the plasma proteins at approximately 7 gm/100 cc of plasma. A decrease in the plasma proteins causes fluid to pass from the blood vessel into the extravascular tissues.

Hyperproteinemia. When the plasma protein rises above 8.5 to 10 gm/100 cc of plasma, the following pathologic conditions may be present: hepatic diseases, toxic conditions, infections and extreme dehydration. Hyperproteinemia occurs in multiple myeloma.

Cloudy Swelling (Parenchymatous Degeneration). Cloudy swelling is a reversible alteration in protein metabolism occurring in mild toxic states. This alteration represents the initial morphologic change seen in an injured cell. The cell imbibes fluid, and protein precipitates from the normal colloidal state forming intracellular granules. Microscopically, the cells appear enlarged, granular and reticulated.

Hydropic Degeneration. Hydropic degeneration is a disturbance manifested in cells as an increase in size because the cells imbibe an excess of water. The cells contain clear vacuoles, composed of water, in their cytoplasm. The nucleus is displaced by the vacuoles. Hydropic degeneration of stratified squamous epithelium is characterized by the presence of large squamous cells with relatively small, irregular, and hyperchromatic nuclei surrounded by transparent cytoplasm. In advanced hydropic degeneration, large cells with clear perinuclear zones occupy a major portion of the epithelium.

Hyaline Change. Hyaline changes are observed in both epithelial and mesenchymal tissues. An irreversible change resulting in the production of a clear translucent protein precipitate similar to the matrix of hyaline cartilage is termed *hyaline degeneration* or *necrosis*.

Hyaline Degeneration (Connective Tissue Hyaline). Hyaline degeneration is seen in old scars and in neoplasms of connective tissue containing a rich collagen component. Lipid material is incorporated into connective tissue hyaline.

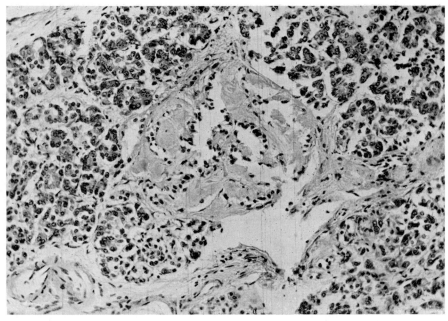

Figure 1. Hyalinization of the pancreatic islets in a case of diabetes mellitus. Notice the hyaline necrosis in the islets of Langerhans of the pancreas. The hyaline material appears morphologically similar to amyloid and may represent a special variety or form of amyloid. Pancreatic acini surround the hyalinized pancreatic islets.

Hyaline Droplet Degeneration (Epithelial Hyaline). Epithelial cells of the body have the capacity to produce a physical hyaline material. In epithelial cells, small to large, homogeneous, deeply eosinophilic droplets may be observed in the cytoplasm associated with degenerative changes.

Zenker's Hyaline Degeneration or Necrosis. Hyaline necrosis may occur in muscle fibers following an aggregation of the sarcoplasm of muscles. This alteration is termed *Zenker's hyaline degeneration* or *necrosis*.

Disturbances in Metabolism of Carbohydrate-Protein (Mucopolysaccharide and Mucoprotein) Complexes

There are two viscid acidic fluids which are formed in epithelial and connective tissues. One material is derived from mesoderm and is termed *mucoid fluid*. Another material is elaborated by epithelial cells and is termed *mucin*.

Disturbances in the Secretion of Mucin. Mucin has a viscid character and is produced in abnormal amounts during pathologic processes. In catarrhal inflammation and most other inflammations there is an increased secretion of mucin. The excretory ducts of salivary glands may become filled with stringy mucin. Neoplasms associated with elaboration of mucin are termed *mucoepidermoid carcinomas*.

Mucoid Change (Myxomatous Connective Tissue). In neoplasms the stroma may show a decrease in cellularity and the intercellular substance

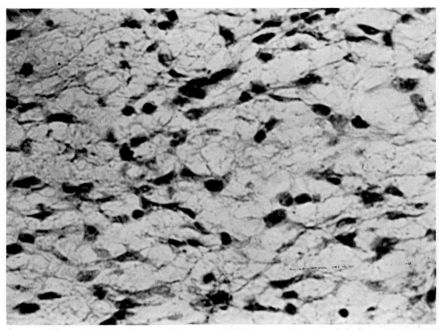

Figure 2. Mucoid change or myxomatous connective tissue. Notice the mucoid or myxomatous material located between cells. The mucoid material is formed by connective tissue.

TABLE I-A

DEGENERATIONS (DEVITALIZATION, REVERSIBLE)

Epithelial	*Mesenchymal*
Cloudy swelling	Mucoid change or mucinolysis (increased water and swelling)
Fatty change	Hyaline droplets in connective
Fatty degeneration	tissue
Fatty metamorphosis	
Fat phanerosis	
Hydropic degeneration	
Mucinous degeneration (epithelial cells)	
Hyaline droplet degeneration	

TABLE I-B

NECROSIS (IRREVERSIBLE)

Coagulation necrosis	Amyloid necrosis
Caseation necrosis *	Fibrinoid necrosis
Liquifaction necrosis	
Hyaline necrosis *	
Fatty necrosis	

* Undergoes dystrophic calcification.

appears as a bluish-gray translucent material. The alteration is termed *mucoid change,* or *myxomatous connective tissue.* The connective tissue in neoplasms may produce myxomatous connective tissue.

Disturbances in the Metabolism of Lipid

Metabolism of Fats in Tissue. The most important lipid is cholesterol. Hypercholesterolemia is associated with pathologic processes. However, future investigations will be required to determine the diagnostic value of high cholesterol in the blood.

Accumulation of Lipids in Reticuloendothelial Cells. Disturbances in the metabolism of lipids are associated with an accumulation of lipids in reticulo-endothelial cells such as cerebroside lipoidosis in Gaucher's disease and phosphatide lipoidosis in Niemann-Pick disease. Reticuloendotheliosis or histiocytosis X result in cholesterol lipoidosis in reticuloendothelial cells. Hand-Schüller-Christian disease is a form of xanthomatosis. Bone destruction may occur and cholesterol-laden phagocytic cells fill the defect.

Fatty Ingrowth. Normal adipose tissue cells filled with visible lipid grow into an adjacent tissue or organ during fatty ingrowth. Fatty ingrowth may rarely occur in the salivary glands resulting in a nonneoplastic swelling of the affected glands. Fatty ingrowth is present in the parotid glands of individuals with malnutrition and inanition and produces a bilateral diffuse enlargement of the parotid glands.

Fatty Change. When lipid enters tissues, fat accumulates within cells due to an accumulation of an excess amount of chemical fat. Fatty change is a reversible abnormal deposition of fat within cells which physiologically contain some invisible fat. The common sites for fatty change are in the liver, kidney and heart.

Wallerian Degeneration. Severance or trauma to nerve trunks and peripheral nerves causes fatty change at the distal segment of the injured nerve. The axon and myelin are converted into tiny droplets and globules of unsaturated fat. This type of fatty change is termed *Wallerian degeneration*.

Progressive Lipodystrophy. Atrophy of subcutaneous fat may occur in the head and neck regions in young females. At the same time, deposition of fat takes place in the lower extremities and buttocks. The subcutaneous tissues of the face and neck become markedly atrophic.

Disturbances in the Absorption of Fat. The failure of absorption of fats results in *intestinal lipodystrophy*. Infants and young children may show a cessation of growth with diarrhea, large whitish frothy fat-laden stools and abdominal distention. The latter findings occur in *celiac disease*. Celiac disease is an infantile form of *sprue*. Sprue is characterized by an impairment of the intestinal absorption of fat and fat-soluble vitamins. The chief signs and symptoms are steatorrhea, loss of weight, hyperchromic macrocytic anemia, hypochlorhydria, sore and/or edematous tongue. Mild cheilosis occurs and the tongue may have an extreme pallor or an intense red, purplish blue or magenta color. In early sprue the tongue has a strawberry appearance.

Glossitis may be the initial symptom of sprue. The tongue becomes extremely sore, painful and fissured. *A peculiar glossitis and stomatitis resulting in a painful, sore and inflamed mouth with a history of diarrhea indicates a tentative diagnosis of sprue.*

Disturbances in the Metabolism of Carbohydrate (Glycogen)

Effects of a Deficiency of Dietary Carbohydrate. If the carbohydrate stores of the liver are depleted, the human organism becomes more susceptible to hepatotoxic agents. Therefore, a patient who is to receive a general anesthetic or is suffering from an infectious disease has a greater chance of re-

TABLE II

FORMS OF TISSUE DEGENERATION (REVERSIBLE, DEVITALIZATION)

EPITHELIAL DEGENERATIONS			MESENCHYMAL DEGENERATIONS
Protein	*Lipid*	*Mucoproteins*	*Mucoproteins*
Cloudy swelling	Fatty change: fatty degeneration fatty metamorphosis fat phanerosis	Mucinous degeneration	Mucinous degeneration (mucoid change)
In mild toxic states epithelial cell imbibes water. Protein precipitates from colloidal state appearing as granules.	In severe toxic states abnormal accumulation of fat droplets occurs in parenchymal cells.	Epithelial tumor cells secrete mucin. Also refers to secretion of mucin, a structureless viscid material secreted by epithelial cells.	Usually occurs in tumors (myxoma). Stroma of connective tissue tumor becomes myxomatous. Increased water and swelling of tissue.
Hydropic degeneration	Fatty ingrowth or stromal fatty infiltration		
Cell imbibes water in great excess. Often seen in renal tubular epithelium after intravenous glucose therapy. Occurs frequently in oral mucosa.	Excessive fat accumulation in stromal connective tissue between parenchymal cells of organs.		
Epithelial hyaline			
Translucent, homogeneous structureless eosin staining physical material of epithelial origin.			
Hyaline droplet degeneration			
In severe injuries eosin staining droplets accumulate in cytoplasm of cell.			

FORMS OF TISSUE NECROSIS (IRREVERSIBLE)

Protein	*Lipid*	*Liquefaction Necrosis*	*Fibrinoid Necrosis*	*Nuclear Damage in Necrosis*
Coagulation necrosis	Caseation necrosis	Necrotic tissue softens and liquifies. Liquification of pus (abscess). Dead cells liberate proteolytic enzymes resulting in self-digestion (autolysis). Caseation necrosis and coagulation necrosis undergo liquefaction necrosis.	Hypersensitivity reaction. Well-defined, clear, translucent, homogeneous to finely granular appearance. Reacts with stains specific for fibrin. Fibrin has been demonstrated in the fibrinoid of some human diseases but not in others.	Pyknosis
Precipitation of proteins including fibrin which resists autolysis.	Toxic avascular "cheesy" necrosis, liberated fatty acids resist autolysis. Undergoes dystrophic calcification. A form of coagulation necrosis in which lipid substances are precipitated.			Shrinkage of nucleus with dense staining reaction in injured cells.
Hyaline necrosis	Gummatous necrosis			Karyorrhexis
Occurs in wide range of connective tissue injuries. Represents replacement of normal structures by amorphous translucent protein precipitate of glassy physi-	Similar to caseation necro-			Fragmentation of nucleus or breaking up of nuclear substance in injured cells.
				Karyolysis
				Fading out or obliteration of nucleus in injured cells.

cal appearance. Undergoes dystrophic calcification.

Amyloidosis

Occurs in chronic infections with tissue destruction. A form of hyalin-like material distinguishable by histochemical staining. An unknown series of protein complex compounds. Hyaline material accumulates between parenchymal cells and in connective tissues. Stains with congo red. Grossly stains with iodine plus sulphuric acid. Grossly anyloid stains with congo red or cresyl violet. Zenkers Hyaline Necrosis: Striated muscle necrosis with replacement of fibers by hyaline change.

sis microscopically, grossly rubbery not cheesy.

Fat necrosis

Splitting of fat; pancreatic lipase which spills into peripherally located fat.

PATHOLOGIC CALCIFICATION

Dystrophic Calcification

Calcium salts are deposited in necrotic tissue.

Metastatic Calcification

Calcium precipitates into normal tissue because of an excess in the circulating blood due to excess parathyroid hormone or in Hypervitaminosis D. Primary organs affected are stomach, lung, thyroid, and kidney.

Calcinosis

Calcium deposited in mesenchymal tissues of the skin. Etiology unknown.

covery if adequate amounts of glucose are administered prior to any surgical procedures.

Hyperglycemia. Diabetes mellitus is the most prominent cause of prolonged hyperglycemia that leads to glycogen infiltrations.

Glycogen Infiltration. During diabetes mellitus the glycogen in storage depots is converted to glucose. Glycogen may be produced in neoplasms particularly in the hypernephroma of the kidney.

Von Gierke's Disease (Glycogen Storage Disease). In Von Gierke's disease large amounts of glycogen are stored in cells and the glycogen cannot be mobilized. Glycogen storage disease is a fatal childhood disease due to a defect in the transformation of glycogen to glucose. Glycogen storage disease may produce *macroglossia.*

Disturbance in the Metabolism of Nucleic Acid

Gout. The joints contain fine, white, irregular foci of sodium urate within the articular cartilages. In advanced gout the articular cartilage may be eroded and the crystalline urate deposit occurs within adjacent bone. *Tophi,* i.e. sodium urate, are present in the cartilagenous lobes of the ears. The blood uric acid is elevated from 3.5 to 6 to 12 mg/100 cc of blood.

Disturbance in the Metabolism of Protein

In a few pathologic conditions abnormal proteins are formed—amyloid and *Bence Jones* protein.

Amyloidosis. Amyloid is a product of a disturbance of protein metabolism. The mechanism of formation of amyloid is unknown.

All organs and tissues may contain amyloid including the gingiva and the tongue. Amyloid causes macroglossia with limitation of function. Amyloid is deposited beneath the endothelium of capillaries and in the walls of arterioles. Amyloid is a pale eosinophilic, extracellular substance with characteristic histochemical properties.

Types of Amyloidosis. There are four distinct types of amyloidosis and they are as follows: (1) primary amyloidosis, (2) secondary amyloidosis, (3) amyloid associated with multiple myeloma and (4) tumor forming amyloid.

Primary amyloidosis involves tissues of mesodermal origin. The most frequent sites of involvement include the intestines, submucosa, myocardium, valves of the heart, larynx, nasal septum, trachea, bronchi, thyroid gland, and smooth and striated muscle. In *secondary amyloidosis* deposits of amyloid occur in the parenchymatous organs associated with a chronic disease. *Amyloidosis associated with multiple myeloma* is another type of amyloidosis. Multiple myeloma is a neoplasm of plasma cells in which tumor-like masses of cells are found in the skeletal system. Hyperproteinemia is present in multiple myeloma. Approximately seven percent of instances of multiple myeloma are associated with primary amyloidosis. *Tumor forming amyloid* is due to the deposition of amyloid in tumor-like nodules in the subcutaneous tissues of the skin.

The mesenchymal tissues involved during amyloidosis show metachromatic staining with methyl violet. The gross specimen from a biopsy will stain red with congo red dye due to an affinity for amyloid. Amyloid affects the blood vessels leading to atrophy and necrosis.

Secondary amyloidosis should always be considered in a differential diagnosis of macroglossia. The amyloid tongue is enlarged, firm, tough and pale. The primary form of amyloidosis may occur in the tongue of healthy individuals. The primary form is rare compared to secondary amyloidosis of the tongue.

Clinical Tests for Amyloidosis. The *congo red test* is a good diagnostic test for amyloid. When an intravenous injection of aqueous congo red is administered to an individual with amyloidosis, the blood level of congo red falls rapidly because amyloid has a great affinity for congo red. In 90 percent of individuals the absorption of congo red by the tissues confirms the diagnosis of amyloidosis.

Bence Jones Protein. Bence Jones protein is found in blood plasma and urine of approximately 70 percent of patients with multiple myeloma.

Tissue Necrosis and Gangrene

Irreversible Cell Damage. Alterations in the form of irreversible damage producing death and decay of cells during life is termed *necrosis*. When disease or injury causes irreversible damage involving the entire organism, the term *somatic death* is used. *Necrobiosis* is the gradual aging and death of cells during life.

Etiology of Necrosis. Tissue necrosis is caused by ischemia or anoxia, malnutrition, pathogenic organisms and their toxins, physical agents and chemical agents.

Morphology of Cells Undergoing Necrosis. In necrotic tissues the cell nucleus becomes small and dense. The latter nuclear change is termed *pyknosis*. When the nucleus ruptures into small fragments the nuclear alteration is termed *karyorrhexis*. Enzymes may split ribonucleic acid and nuclear protein, causing a swelling of the nucleus, loss of chromatin, and dissolution of the nucleus. The latter nuclear change is termed *karyolysis*.

Individual Forms of Necrosis and Gangrene

Coagulation Necrosis. Coagulation necrosis occurs whenever the protoplasm of a cell undergoes an abrupt coagulation of protein. Histologically, the necrotic tissue has a distinct outline and the cell outlines remain intact. *Infarction* is coagulation necrosis of tissues following complete blockage of the blood supply. In early infarction the cell outlines persist.

Caseation Necrosis. Caseation necrosis is a process of cell death produced by tubercle bacilli. The necrotic tissue consists of a granular soft and friable mass of coagulated protein and fat. Microscopically, there is a complete absence of tissue architecture.

Gummatous Necrosis. Gummatous necrosis of the palate occurs in terti-

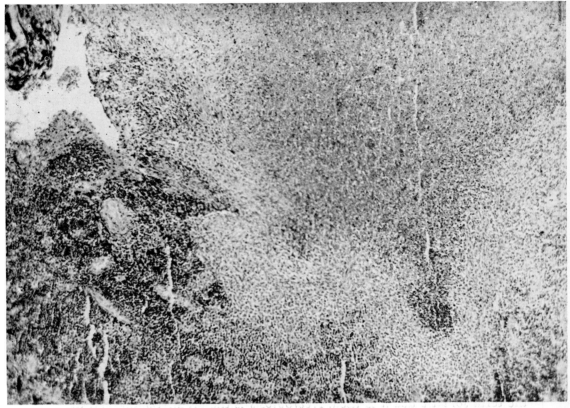

Figure 3. Caseation necrosis. Notice the structureless mass of coagulative necrotic tissue in the center of a tubercle. No blood vessels are present in the zone of caseation necrosis. Lymphocytes border the periphery of the zone of caseation necrosis.

ary syphilis. Gummas heal by absorption of the necrotic material and fibrosis.

Liquefaction Necrosis. Liquefaction necrosis is the result of autolytic enzymes which are abundant in necrotic tissues. Necrotic tissue is rapidly decomposed, and is surrounded by liquified material. Suppuration is a form of liquefaction necrosis.

Fat Necrosis. Necrosis of fat is irreversible death of fatty tissue due to pancreatic disease.

Fibrinoid Necrosis. Fibrinoid necrosis is an irreversible collagen alteration composed of eosinophilic deposits with some characteristics of fibrin. Fibrinoid necrosis produces a highly refractile, irregular, eosinophilic material forming coarsely reticular structures or solid homogeneous masses in the extracellular tissues.

Gangrene (Wet and Dry Forms). Gangrene is a massive form of tissue necrosis. The necrosis consists of death of tissue plus putrefaction—a super-imposed saprophytic bacterial infection. A blue, black or green color occurs and a foul odor results from the ingress of saprophytic and gas forming organisms into the necrotic tissue. The dry form of gangrene is an infarct-coagulation necrosis. Wet gangrene is necrosis plus invasion by saprophytic organisms. Senile gangrene is necrosis in an extremity, i.e. dry gangrene due to arteriosclerosis. Diabetic gangrene is due to arteriosclerosis but occurs much earlier than senile gangrene. Gangrene of the cheeks is termed *noma*. Noma is due to an anaerobic fusospirochetal infection producing a gangrenous stomatitis in debilitated children. Noma is a rapidly progressive gan-

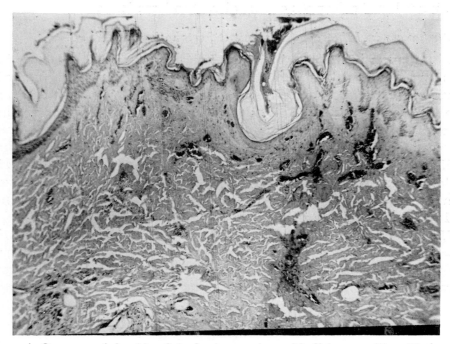

Figure 4. Gangrene of the skin of the leg in a patient with diabetes mellitus. Notice the massive necrosis of the skin which has been invaded by saprophytic microorganisms. The gangrene occurs secondarily following the disturbed metabolism.

grene which begins in the epithelium, spreads to the musculature and perforates the cheek causing extensive tissue discoloration.

Disturbances in the Metabolism of Calcium

Pathologic Calcification. Dystrophic calcification occurs in an area which has previously been the site of tissue necrosis. The blood level of calcium and phosphorus is normal. Dystrophic calcification may occur in the walls of blood vessels following regressive changes. The etiology and pathogenesis of dystrophic calcification are obscure.

Metastatic Calcification. This is characterized by the deposition of calcium salts in tissues which are not the site of regressive change. Metastatic calcification follows a sequel of well-defined pathologic states which leads to a disturbance in calcium and phosphorus metabolism. Metastatic calcification is due to hyperparathyroidism, renal insufficiency, hypervitaminosis D, metastatic carcinoma, multiple myeloma, infantile idiopathic hypercalcemia, and immobilization.

Calcinosis is a special type of pathologic calcification which has an obscure etiology. In adults calcinosis may occur in a localized form limited to an area of the extremities adjacent to the joints. This form of calcinosis is termed *calcinosis circumscripta*. When calcium nodules occur in the fingers, the calcinosis is termed *calcium arthritis*. *Calcinosis universalis* is encountered in children and adolescents. The calcium deposits are numerous, large, and located in the deep structures adjacent to large joints.

Disturbances in Mineral and Pigment Metabolism

Disturbances in the Metabolism of Iron. A disturbance of metabolism resulting in increased iron in the form of pigments in all tissues of the body is termed *hemochromatosis*. In hemochromatosis iron deposition occurs in hepatic cells, Kupffer's cells, the portal triad, and in bile duct proliferations. The triad of diabetes, bronzed skin and cirrhosis of the liver occurs in hemochromatosis.

Hemochromatosis is accompanied by the following features: it occurs in males; the skin contains iron pigment; the spleen is enlarged; the heart contains iron pigment; the pancreas shows fibrosis and diabetes; and the adrenal and pituitary glands are rich in iron pigment.

Hemosiderosis is an excessive deposition of hemosiderin pigment in organs and tissues due to an excessive breakdown of blood. Iron is found in Kupffer's cells and extremely small quantities are present in the connective tissue stroma of the liver and kidney. The serum iron is elevated

TABLE III
PIGMENTS

Exogenous Pigments	*Endogenous Pigments*
Carotene (carotenemia)	Melanin
Reduced silver (argyria)	Ochronosis
Bismuth	Bilirubin
Lead (plumbism)	Derived from hemoglobin
Tattoo	Hemosiderin
Coal (anthracotic pigment)	Polymer of $Fe(OH)_x$ de-
Anthrasilicosis	rived from heme, generally
Siderosis	found in macrophages
Lipochrome	Hematoidin
Considered an exogenous	Myoglobin
pigment	Pigmentation in Brown atrophy
Pneumoconiosis (inhaled dust)	of the heart
	Malarial pigment
	Related to hematin
	Lipofuscin pigment
	Hemofuscin pigment
	In degenerated and necrotic
	hepatic cells

Pigmentations	
Metallic pigments	Melanosis aurea
Lead, mercury, bismuth	Porphyria
amalgam	Lupus erythematosus
Idiopathic pigmentation	Nevus-melanoma
Chloasma	Osler-Weber-Rendu disease
Addison's disease	Neurofibromatosis
Oral melanosis	Stannous fluoride
Albright's syndrome	Tetracyclines
Erythroblastosis fetalis	Vitiligo
Osteitis fibrosa cystica	

when the tissue stores are increased. The body is frozen in its intake and output of iron during hemosiderosis. In idiopathic hemochromatosis the skin becomes pigmented and iron is deposited in the salivary glands.

Exogenous Pigmentation

Pneumoconiosis (Inhaled Dust). Inhalation of dust is termed *pneumoconiosis*. Deposition of carbon pigment in tissues is termed *anthracosis*. Tar containing a high content of carbon passes into the alveolar spaces of the lungs and is taken up by histiocytic cells. Deposition of silica in tissues is termed *silicosis*. Asbestos deposition in tissues is termed *asbestosis*. Inhalation of *iron dust* produces pigmentation of the lungs and pulmonary lymph nodes.

Lead (Plumbism). Lead enters the body through the gastrointestinal and respiratory systems and is deposited around blood vessels and beneath epithelium. Anemia characterized by stippled red blood cells occurs in chronic plumbism.

Reduced Silver (Argyrosis). Argyrosis resulting from silver nitrate medication produces a blue pigmentation in the skin. Silver is deposited in the intercellular tissue, basement membrane and adjacent connective tissue.

Carrot Pigment (Carotenemia). Pigmentation results from an excess of carrots in the diet. When carotenemia occurs, a high concentration of vitamin A is present in the blood. The face, especially the nasolabial folds, palms and soles are pigmented a yellow color.

Endogenous Pigmentation

Melanosis. Melanin pigment appears in lentigo (freckles) and pigmented moles (nevi), Addison's disease, and melanosis coli.

Melanosis Coli. When melanin pigmentation occurs in the mucous membrane of the colon, the condition is termed *melanosis coli*.

Pigmentation in Brown Atrophy of the Heart. The deposition of pigment granules around the nucleus of cardiac fibers is termed *brown atrophy of the heart*.

Ochronosis. Ochronosis is a rare disturbance in endogenous melanin pigmentation. A black discoloration occurs in cartilage, connective tissue, muscle and epithelial cells.

Hematogenous Pigmentations. Pigments derived from hemoglobin arise from the heme portion of the hemoglobin molecule. The iron oxide portion is *hemosiderin* and the derivatives of the porphyrin portion are *hematoporphyrin* and *bilirubin*. *Hematoidin* occurs when hemoglobin is split pathologically into an iron-free hematoidin. Bilirubin is chemically similar to hematoidin and is formed by the breakdown of hemoglobin. Bilirubin is a yellow bile pigment.

Porphyrins. The breakdown of large amounts of hemoglobin results in increased excretion of protoporphyrin in the urine and feces. Porphyrins have a red color and may cause an acquired or congenital disease. Porphyrinemia produces a reddish color to the conjunctiva, skin, bones and urine.

Malarial Pigmentation. The malarial parasite within the red blood cell produces a black colored hematin pigment. The freed black pigment is deposited in the abdominal organs.

Chloasma. Chloasma is a pigmentary disturbance characterized by the appearance of brown patches in the skin of the face and other areas of the body.

Chapter 3

CIRCULATORY DISTURBANCES

EDEMA AND TRANSUDATION

Edema Producing Factors

Edema **Due to Increased Hydrostatic Pressure.** Edema is present during cardiac failure because the return of fluid to the vessels cannot take place. In *edema of cardiac failure* the protein content and specific gravity of the edema fluid are low; therefore, the fluid is termed a *transudate*. The difference between the colloidal osmotic pressure and the hydrostatic pressure at the venous end of the capillary is not great enough to cause the return of fluid to the vessels; therefore, *hypoproteinemic edema* results. *Nephrotic edema* occurs in renal disease with a continuous loss of protein from the plasma into the urine.

Malnutrition causes a low protein level in the blood. During malnutrition, edema occurs in the legs accompanied by ascites, i.e. edema fluid in the abdominal cavity. The total endothelial surface of the lungs is very great. Damage to these endothelial surfaces results in *edema due to increased capillary permeability*.

Character of the Edema Fluid

Extravascular fluid poor in protein is termed *noninflammatory edema fluid* or a *transudate*. A transudate has a low protein component and low specific gravity. An *exudate* is inflammatory edema fluid. The specific gravity of an exudate is greater than 1.015, may be 1.027, and the protein content is greater than 4 gm/100 ml of fluid.

Complications of Edema

Serous edema fluid in the tissues leads to secondary infection. The function of the tissue is impaired by the presence of edema. When edema produces an obstruction to the air passage a serious complication is present.

BLOOD CLOTTING MECHANISM

The intrinsic blood clotting mechanism relates to the formation of the fibrin clot within the intact vascular system. The Hageman factor (XII) in the plasma is activated by surface contact to activated Hageman factor. This reaction occurs at a slow rate. The activated Hageman factor is the catalyst responsible for conversion of plasma thromboplastic antecedent (PTA or factor XI) into the activated factor XI. The activated factor XI plus calcium are responsible for the conversion of plasma thromboplastic component (PTC or factor IX or Christmas factor) into activated factor IX. Activated factor IX plus calcium are responsible for conversion of antihemophilic globulin (AGH or factor VIII) into activated factor VIII. Activated factor VIII plus calcium convert the Stuart-Prower factor (factor X) into activated factor X. At this stage the reaction is becoming more rapid. Activated factor X converts proaccelerin (factor V) into activated factor V. Activated factor V plus platelet factor 3 yield thromboplastin (factor III). Thromboplastin (factor III) plus calcium and platelet factor 2 convert prothrombin (factor II) into thrombin. At this stage the reaction is rapid. Thrombin plus calcium and platelet factor I are responsible for the conversion of fibrinogen (factor I) into fibrin monomer. Fibrin monomer is responsible for the conversion of fibrin polymer into a soluble fibrin clot. At this stage the reaction is explosive in nature. The fibrin stabilizing factor (factor XIII or fibrinase or Laki-Lorand factor) is responsible for the conversion of the soluble fibrin clot to the insoluble fibrin gel.

In the extrinsic blood clotting mechanism tissue thromboplastin, proconvertin (factor VII), proaccelerin (factor V), and the Stuart-Prower factor (X) plus calcium and platelet factor 2 convert prothrombin (factor II) into thrombin. Thrombin plus calcium and platelet factor I are responsible for conversion of fibrinogen (factor I) into fibrin monomer. Fibrin monomer is responsible for conversion of fibrin polymer into a soluble fibrin clot. The fibrin stabilizing factor (XIII) is responsible for conversion of the soluble fibrin clot into the insoluble fibrin gel.

Hematologic Tests for Diagnostic Purposes

Bleeding time is a function of platelet adequacy. If the bleeding time is greater than fifteen minutes it is considered abnormal. Clotting time is a measure of the adequacy of the thrombin used. A clot retraction evaluation is used as a measure of the adequacy of the blood clot. A platelet count reveals the same information. The circulating anticoagulant test is useful for determining the deficiency of the labile factors. A low prothrombin time produces a deficiency of labile factors. The prothrombin consumption test is a labile factor test utilized during disease states. In hemophilia the individual does not use up all of the available thrombin. Thromboplastinogen is not activated and thus absent because thrombin is not produced. The lack of thrombin causes delayed clot formation. The normal prothrombin consumption time (PCT) is twelve seconds. In the hemophiliac the PCT is twelve to thirteen seconds. The prothrombin time is a test used to measure the clotting efficiency of blood. Normally clotting takes place in ten to twelve seconds. The normal prothrombin time (PT) of the serum after clotting is fifteen seconds. In hemophiliacs the PT is eight to ten seconds, which is lower than the PT value before clotting. The platelets and bleeding time are normal in hemophilia. In thrombocytopenia the platelets are low and a prolonged bleeding time occurs. Clot retraction evaluation is another useful measure of clot adequacy. Platelet counts are useful as a function of the bleeding time. The activity of platelets may be measured by the thromboplastin activity time.

HEMORRHAGE

Morphologic Changes Resulting from Hemorrhage

When blood escapes into the tissues macrophages, polymorphonuclear leukocytes and lymphocytes mobilize in the area with subsequent fibrosis. Pigmentation is elaborated from the destruction of red blood cells. *Petechiae* and *ecchymosis* are small and moderate hemorrhages in the tissues. *Hematomas* are large hemorrhages generally located in the subcutaneous tissues.

When rapid loss of blood occurs, the blood pressure falls, and syncope and shock develop. The volume of blood decreases during hemorrhage. The spleen contracts, provides blood to the circulation, and a redistribution of blood occurs. Fluid passes from the interstitial compartment into the vessel; therefore, hemodilution takes place.

Causes of Hemorrhage

Hemorrhage is caused by rupture of blood vessel walls due to trauma or pathologic processes. In ulcers the arteries of the lamina propria are subjected to irritation, trauma and infection resulting in hemorrhage. Vitamin C deficiency produces hemorrhage due to capillary damage. The cement substance of capillaries is altered during vitamin C deficiency with hemorrhages occurring in the skin and oral mucosa. The capillary fragility test is a useful indicator of the state of capillaries. If a patient has capillary fragility, petechial hemorrhages occur in the skin. Ecchymosis and petechiae occur in the skin and gingiva during scurvy and leukemia.

Protective Mechanisms Following Hemorrhage. The contraction of vessel walls, the elasticity of vessel walls, the folding of the severed intima, and the slowing of the blood flow are hemostatic protective mechanisms.

THROMBOSIS

Thrombosis is the occlusion of a blood vessel or the presence of a mass in the heart chamber derived from constituents of the circulating blood during life. Thrombosis is a defensive mechanism which seals the blood vessels against loss of blood.

Formation of the Thrombus

Thrombosis is due to stasis of blood, to a change in the composition of the blood, and to endothelial impairment. The endothelium becomes anoxic and the blood platelets adhere to vessel walls. When the viscosity of the blood is increased during stress, the blood flow is decreased and the fibrinogen content of the blood is increased. Increased stickiness of blood platelets occurs when the viscosity is increased. Microscopically, thrombi consist of fibrin, white blood cells, red blood cells and blood platelets all entrapped within a meshwork. Intracardiac thrombi occur on the heart valves and are termed *vegetations*.

Factors Predisposing to Thrombus Formation. A lesion of the endothelium, arteriosclerosis or phlebitis, and changes in the velocity, character and constituents of the blood stream predisposes the blood vessels to thrombosis. In diabetes mellitus disturbances occur in lipid metabolism with subsequent formation of thrombosis.

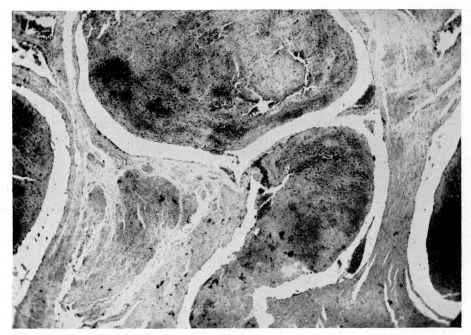

Figure 5. Multiple thrombi in the esophageal wall. Notice the organization occurring in the multiple thrombi. The thrombi are invaded by connective tissue at the sites of adherence to the vessel wall.

Fate of the Thrombus

Organization. Red blood cells in the thrombus are lysed and hemoglobin is broken down into heme. The next step is vascularization of the thrombus. Recanalization follows vascularization. Recanalization reestablishes the circulation with the rest of the body. The calcified thrombotic vein is termed *phlebolith*.

EMBOLISM

The dislodgement of a thrombus either partially or completely starts the mass downstream with eventual occlusion of a smaller caliber vessel. The dislodged mass which occludes a blood vessel is termed an *embolus*. Embo-

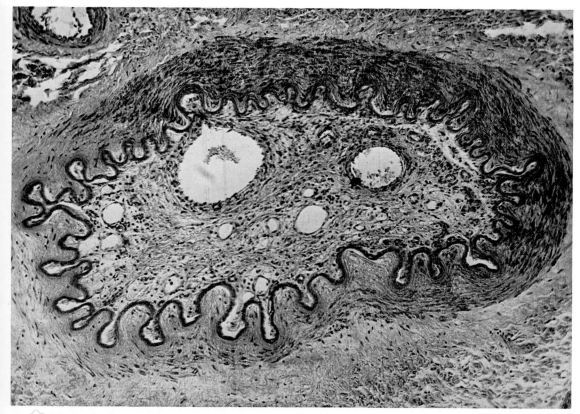

Figure 6. Organization and recanalization of an arterial thrombus. Notice that the re-canalization has taken place in the connective tissue inside of the internal elastic lamina and not in the outer wall of the artery. The dark, broad, wavy line is the internal elastic lamina of the original artery. Organization of the thrombus by fibrous connective tissue and capillaries precedes the recanalization.

lism produces infarcts in organs with a single blood supply. Embolism is rare in organs with a double blood supply, i.e. liver and lungs.

Types of Emboli

A *retrograde embolus* moves against the current of the circulating blood such as the tumor cell embolus. Thrombi produce *thrombotic emboli*. Emboli may be due to fat in the region of fractured bones. The fat enters the severed capillaries and *fat emboli* terminate in the capillaries of the lungs.

Air embolus occurs in the veins of the chest or neck when a negative pressure is present during inspiration. People working under high atmospheric pressures may develop *Caisson disease*. If an individual is decompressed rapidly, carbon dioxide, hydrogen and nitrogen pass to a gaseous state within the blood stream as air embolism. *Tumor cell emboli* may lodge in veins. Tumor cells invade and proliferate in the lumen after passing through the thin wall of veins. Amniotic fluid may be squeezed into veins after a difficult labor forming the *amniotic fluid embolism*. *Bacterial embo-*

lism is produced by colonies of bacteria in the blood stream. A *foreign body embolus* is produced when a foreign body is displaced into an artery.

ISCHEMIA

Ischemia develops in tissues because of thrombosis, hemorrhage, embolism and anoxia. Ischemia is a decrease of the blood flow to the tissues. Raynaud's disease producing gangrene of the fingers is an example of ischemia plus infarction. Atherosclerosis with narrowing of the lumen of blood vessels results in ischemia.

INFARCTION

Embolism and arteriosclerosis cause infarction in tissues and organs with a single circulation. Infarcts do not occur in organs with a double circulation or if anastomoses are present. In organs with a terminal circulation the infarcted area contains a minimal amount of blood, i.e. *ischemic infarct*. *Hemorrhagic infarcts* occur in the lungs because of the double circulation. The fate of an infarct includes organization of the infarct with scar formation, abscess, cyst and gangrene formation.

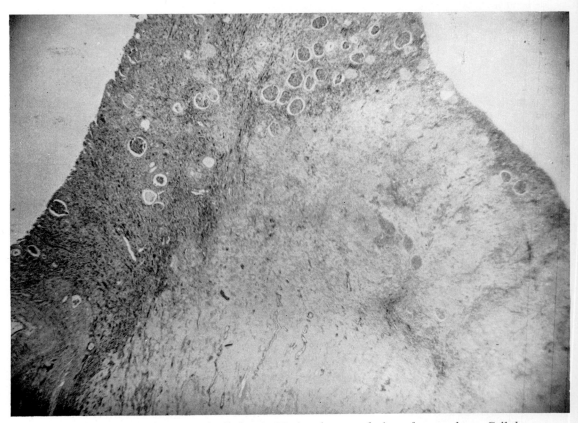

Figure 7. Coagulation necrosis (infarct). Notice the coagulation of protoplasm. Cellular details and, in this instance, some architectural features are absent. In early instances of coagulation necrosis the tissue architecture is preserved. There is a rather sharp delineation between the necrotic and vital tissue.

HYPEREMIA

Active Hyperemia. Active hyperemia is an increase in the amount of blood in the tissues due to dilatation of arterioles and capillaries. An increased amount of blood passes through the tissue because many additional capillaries are utilized.

Passive Hyperemia. Passive hyperemia is due to venous stasis. In passive hyperemia an increased amount of blood is present in the tissues; however, the volume of blood that passes into the tissues per minute is either normal or decreased.

SHOCK

Shock is a clinical syndrome which results from a reduction in the volume of the circulating blood. When hemorrhage is a complication the individual may go into shock.

Primary Shock. Severe pain following an injury produces rapid vasodilatation. After an emotional shock a vasovagal syndrome may occur in which the individual has general vasodilatation. Blood drains away from the brain to the dependent parts and cerebral anoxia results. Low blood pressure is present with slow pulse, pale face, sweat and cold extremities. This state can be reversed rapidly by placing the individual in a supine position. Primary shock is temporary neurogenic shock—a neurovascular state which cannot be differentiated from *syncope*.

Secondary Shock. Secondary shock takes place secondary to some situation. Clinically, a wound of fairly extensive size is present. The patient has the following symptoms: low blood pressure, fast pulse, cold skin over the extremities, thirst, dyspnea, sweating and loss of blood externally from the wound and internally into the tissues.

Pathophysiology of Shock. The initial circulatory change in shock is a decrease in blood volume and reduced blood pressure in the aorta and systemic arteries. The decreased blood pressure in the aorta is responsible for initiating the adaptive reflex in the aortic arch resulting in a generalized vasoconstriction. The carotid sinus reflex follows the lowered aortic blood pressure resulting in an increased heart rate. Vasoconstriction results in the release of blood to the vital organs.

Kinds of Shock. In *wound shock* loss of blood occurs externally and internally in the region of injury. Wound shock is associated with decreased circulating blood volume. In *hemorrhagic shock* loss of blood occurs on the surface of the skin or into the gastrointestinal tract. In *burn shock,* a variant of wound or hemorrhagic shock, a loss of fluid exudate occurs in the area of the burn.

Crush Syndrome. The crush syndrome follows severe burns of the extremities. The tissues become edematous with decreased blood volume when the crushing pressure is relieved. The damaged capillaries permit the seepage of fluid and the individual passes into shock.

TABLE IV

DIFFERENTIATING FEATURES OF SECONDARY
SHOCK AND HEMORRHAGE

	Secondary Shock	*Hemorrhage*
Endothelium	Permeable to colloids	Impermeable
Flow of lymph	Increased	Decreased
Tissue fluid	Increased	Decreased
Fluid balance	Disturbed	Undisturbed
Vomiting	Persistent	None
Diarrhea	Frequent	Absent
Renal		
Excretions	Deficient or decreased	Low volume
Urine	Concentrated	No change
	Low volume, albumen, erythrocytes, bile	
	Debris	
Blood		
Coagulation time	Increased	Decreased
Concentration	Increased	Decreased
NPN	Increased	Unchanged
Plasma Na and Plasma chloride	Decreased	Unchanged
K	Increased	Terminal increase
Blood sugar	Increased	Increased
Necropsy findings		
Edema of soft tissue	Characteristic	None
Serious effusions	Present	Absent
Capillovenous congestion	Characteristic	Absent
Petechiae	Characteristic	Absent
Visceral ischemia	Absent	Present
Organ weight	Increased	Decreased
GI tract	Congested, dilated, atonic	Contracted
Parenchymal necrosis	Present	Absent

TABLE V

SHOCK SEQUENCE

1. Fluid loss or blood loss
2. Hypotension
3. Reduced venous return to the right heart
4. Renal ischemia
5. Progressive hypotension
6. Hemoconcentration
7. Lower nephron nephrosis
8. Massive circulatory collapse

Chapter 4

PRINCIPLES OF INFLAMMATION, REGENERATION AND REPAIR

INTRODUCTION, DEFINITION AND CAUSES OF INFLAMMATION

Inflammation is the basis of all body responses. The tissues of the body are capable of responding with a local dynamic mechanism to counteract irritants. The response of tissues to an injury is termed *inflammation*. Every tissue and organ of the human body is capable of responding to an injury or irritant by the same dynamic mechanism termed *inflammation*. The causative agents of injury to all tissues may be of endogenous origin, i.e. necrosis and gangrene due to vascular disturbances. Disturbances in metabolic processes provoke inflammation. The causative agents of injury may be of exogenous origin. Inflammation is a highly complex vascular, lymphatic and local reaction of tissue to an irritant or injury. Inflammation has beneficial effects because it dilutes, neutralizes, localizes, and removes the irritant causing the injury.

PRINCIPLES OF STARLING'S HYPOTHESIS

Transport of Molecules Across Membranes. Starling * proposed the hypothesis that water and electrolytes would readily pass through the capillary wall; however, the plasma proteins were unable to escape and therefore remained within the capillaries. Exchanges of fluid according to Starling's hypothesis are relatively limited. The difference between the hydrostatic pressure and the osmotic pressure of the plasma is more important for maintaining the blood volume than for producing the exchanges of fluid between the capillaries and the tissues. Diffusion through the endothelial cell plays the major role in the transportation of molecules across the capillary wall. In inflammation an increase in the number of opened capillaries accounts for the redness of the tissues. The increased hydrostatic pressure is one reason for an increase in the quantity of fluid passing out of capillaries into the extravascular spaces. Damaged endothelium is likewise responsible for increased fluid leaving the capillaries. This movement of fluid is aided by increased permeability of capillary walls. The higher the venous hydrostatic pressure, the less the quantity of fluid returning to the blood stream.

---

* Starling, E. H.: Tissue fluid formation and absorption: *J Physiol* (London), *19:* 312, 1895–1896.

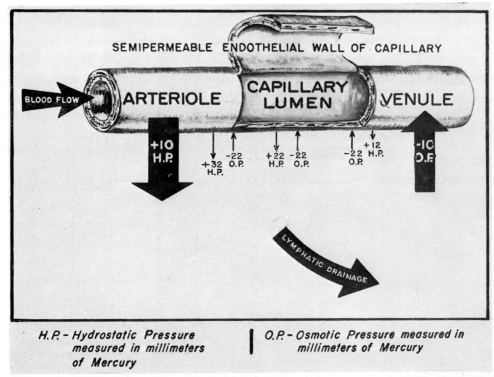

Figure 8. Diagrammatic representation of the passage of water and electrolytes out of an arteriole and returning to a venule according to Starling's Hypothesis.

ACTIVE TRANSPORT AND PINOCYTOSIS

Active transport takes place when energy, originating from the metabolism of cells, causes the movement of substances across the cell membrane. Many cells obtain substances within the cell membrane by pinocytosis (cell drinking) or by phagocytosis (cell eating). Pinocytosis is not an alternative to membrane transport, but is rather a supporting mechanism.

CAPILLARY STRUCTURE

The capillary wall consists of a single cellular layer—the endothelium. The permeability of the capillary wall is due to pores which occupy a small part of the total surface of the wall. A double pathway occurs across the capillary wall, i.e. by way of the endothelial cell for lipid-soluble substances. Vesicles located in the endothelium may transport water and solutes across the endothelial cell proper.

CAUSES OF CAPILLARY PERMEABILITY IN INFLAMMATION

Histamine. Histamine is a substance capable of increasing permeability of the capillary wall during inflammation. The lesion produced by histamine is a local discontinuity in the endothelium caused by the separation of two adjacent endothelial cells.

Leukotaxine and Peptides. Menkin * isolated a capillary permeability factor from the inflammatory exudate which he termed *leukotaxine*.

Exudin. Exudin is a substance released by injured cells and is probably related to the peptides.

Necrosin. Menkin * concluded that a toxic euglobulin is liberated by injured cells at the site of the irritant. He designated the euglobulin as necrosin.

Nucleotides and Nucleosides. Several nucleosides and the nucleotide inosinic acid are responsible for altered capillary permeability during inflammation.

Five-hydroxytryptamine. Five-hydroxytryptamine is present in inflammation increasing capillary permeability only in the earliest stage of inflammation.

Permeability Globulin Factor. Increased capillary permeability is due to an a_1 globulin. The a_1 globulin is termed the *permeability globulin factor*.

BASIC REACTIONS OF TISSUES TO IRRITANTS AND INJURY

Sequence of Events in the Inflammatory Response. The basic response of inflammation is a dynamic series of alterations which are initiated by hu-

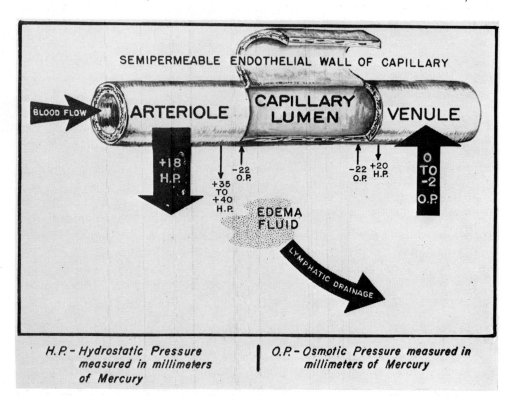

Figure 9. Diagrammatic representation of the passage of increased fluid and plasma proteins through a capillary in an area of inflammation. Edema fluid accumulates in the tissues in the manner illustrated in this diagram.

* Menkin, V.: *Biochemical Mechanisms in Inflammation.* Springfield, Thomas, 1956.

moral substances which exert their effect on the local vascular system. The sequence of events is as follows: (1) transient vasoconstriction followed by dilatation of arterioles, (2) increased blood flow through arterioles, capillaries and venules, (3) capillary dilatation and increased permeability of the capillary wall, (4) passage of transudate through permeable capillary wall, (5) increase in number of red blood cells per unit area of capillaries, (6) slowing or complete stasis of blood, (7) margination of white blood cells, (8) passage of inflammatory exudate through permeable capillary walls and (9) passage of white blood cells from capillaries (polymorphonuclear leukocytes first, followed by monocytes, lymphocytes and plasma cells).

Vascular Responses and Fluid Exudation in Inflammation. A temporary vasoconstriction of arterioles is the earliest vascular response in inflammation. The transient vasoconstriction is rapidly followed by vasodilatation. The vasodilatation is due to the direct action of the humoral substances on the walls of the arterioles and by local axon reflexes. The humoral agents have the capacity to alter the endothelium of the dilated arterioles producing sticky endothelial cells and a permeable arteriole.

Due to the change in the size of the affected vessels and the increased permeability there is a transudation of fluid from the altered vessels. The viscosity of the blood is increased resulting in a slowing of the blood stream in the affected blood vessels. When slowing or stasis occurs, the white blood cells are attracted to the periphery. With decreased movement of blood the polymorphonuclear leukocytes adhere to the sticky endothelial cells. In a few hours the white blood cells line up along the endothelium of the vessels. The latter is termed *margination or pavementation.*

Fluid Responses and Exudation in Inflammation. In burns, sunburn and liquid burns, vesicles composed of serous exudates form rapidly in the tissues. Within minutes a serous exudate is present. When a severe injury occurs in tissues, permeability and porosity of the vessel wall increases so that the larger molecules may pass out of the vessels.

Cellular Responses and Exudation in Inflammation. The process of *emigration* follows margination. By pseudopod movement, the polymorphonuclear leukocytes migrate between the endothelial cells. By ameboid movement the leukocytes pass through the vessel wall into the extravascular spaces. The polymorphonuclear leukocytes are the most dominant cells in acute inflammation. Monocytes migrate through the altered vessel wall at a much slower rate than polymorphonuclear leukocytes. If inflammation is rampant, red blood cells may pass through the capillary wall by *rhexis.* During rhexis the capillary wall is broken at one point and red blood cells pass out of the vessel. Red blood cells and white blood cells also pass through the capillary wall by *diapedesis.*

Bacteria, tissue debris, albumins, globulins and fibrinogens all may take part in aiding the migrating cells to move away from the blood vessels in a well-directed fashion. This well-directed movement of cells away from the blood vessels directly to the injured tissue is a chemotactic one and the process is termed *chemotaxis*.

CELLULAR ELEMENTS IN THE INFLAMMATORY EXUDATE

Polymorphonuclear Leukocytes

The *neutrophilic leukocyte* is the most important cell mobilized in tissues injured by invading pyogenic organisms. The dead and dying leukocytes represent the pathognomonic cellular element in suppuration. The function of the neutrophile is phagocytosis or pinocytosis and the production of proteolytic enzymes.

The precise function of the *eosinophile* is obscure. The presence of the *mast cell* during inflammation has been interpreted as a sign of healing.

Mononuclear Leukocytes

Lymphocytes are present in tissues during subacute and chronic inflammation and during healing. Their function is unknown. *Plasma cells* are related to lymphocytes and their function is antibody formation. *Monocytes* from the blood and *macrophages* arising in the tissues are of a single cell type.

LOCAL CLINICAL FEATURES OF INFLAMMATION

Cardinal Signs of Inflammation. The five cardinal signs of inflammation are rubor or redness, calor or heat, tumor or swelling, dolor or pain and *functio laesa* or disturbed function. Redness and heat are due to an increase in the amount of blood in the injured tissue. Swelling is due to the passage of fluid and cells from the capillaries into the interstitial spaces with a diminished return of fluid to the venous end of the capillary. Pain is due to the increased pressure acting upon nerves resulting in a stimulation of both sensory and motor nerve endings. The interference with function is voluntary or is due to the exudate stimulating sensory and motor nerve endings.

Lymphatic Blockage in Tissues. Pyogenic microorganisms which provoke inflammation are capable of causing a fibrin thrombus in the local lymphatics. Lymphatic blockage is rapidly produced in response to staphylococci.

SYSTEMIC EFFECTS OF INFLAMMATION

The systemic effects include changes in the circulating blood stream leading to a leukocytosis at the expense of the polymorphonuclear leukocytes.

PURPOSE OF THE INFLAMMATORY EXUDATE

Function of Elements that Pass into the Tissues During Inflammation. The functions of the natural antibodies and properidin which are present in the inflammatory exudate are detoxification, dilution and localization of the irritant. Antibodies are carried to the site of injury by gamma globulin.

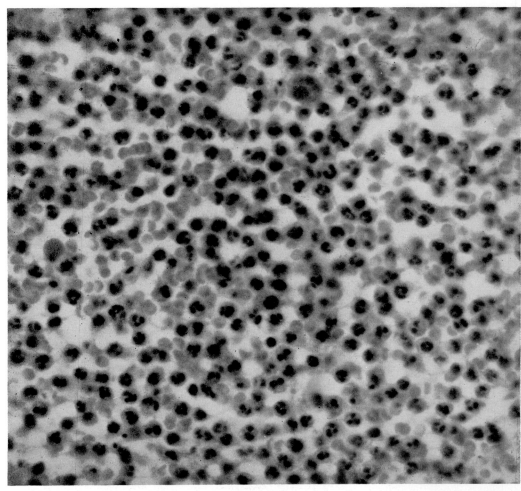

Figure 10. Acute inflammation. Notice the dense infiltrate composed entirely of polymorphonuclear leukocytes.

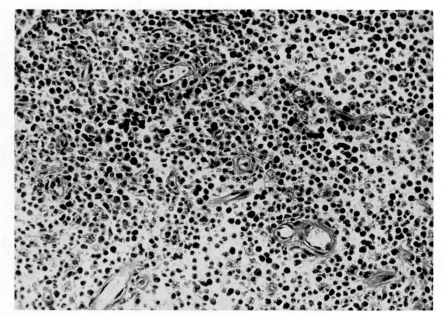

Figure 11. Abscess. Notice the purulent exudate (pus) which consists of dead or dying polymorphonuclear leukocytes and necrotic material. This abscess has been walled off by fibrous connective tissue.

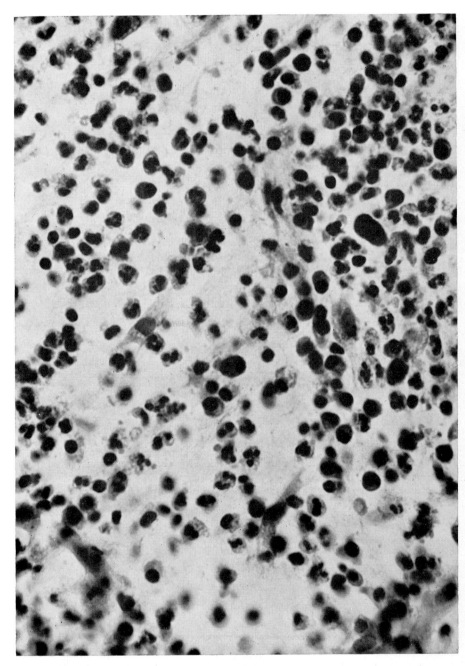

Figure 12. Subacute inflammation. Notice the numerous polymorphonuclear leukocytes interspersed among plasma cells and lymphocytes.

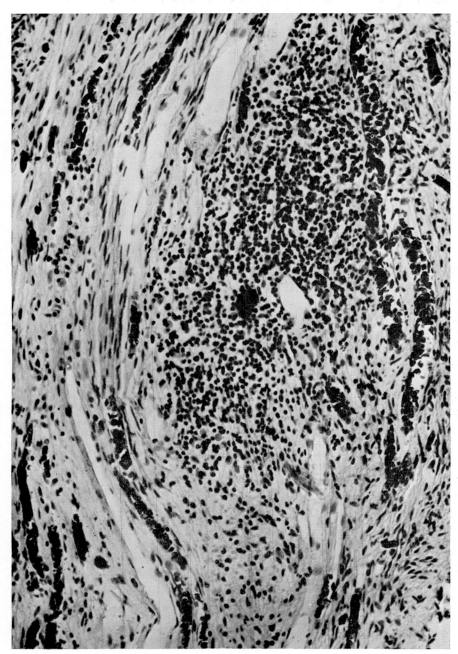

Figure 13. Chronic inflammation. Notice the dense infiltrate composed almost entirely of small lymphocytes. The cytoplasm of the lymphocyte is minimal and therefore not readily visualized in tissue sections. Plasma cells and mononuclear phagocytes may accompany lymphocytes in chronic inflammation.

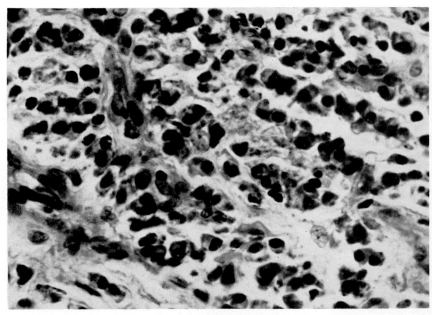

Figure 14. Chronic inflammation. Notice that the predominant cell in this case of chronic inflammation is the plasma cell. Lymphocytes and macrophages are also common in chronic inflammation. Polymorphonuclear leukocytes are absent or rare during chronic inflammation.

The fluid portion of the exudate contains sodium, potassium, sulphate, phosphate and carbonate.

CLINICAL CORRELATION OF INFLAMMATION

Abscess. An abscess is a circumscribed collection of pus. It may occur in the tissues and cause destruction and resorption of bone or it may occur in the skin and lips. The affected area becomes infiltrated with a mass of polymorphonuclear leukocytes which die, producing pus. Pus may be sterile, i.e. consist of liquified necrotic cells which are free of bacteria.

Boil—Carbuncle. A boil is an abscess of a hair follicle. When fusion of boils occurs a carbuncle results.

Sinus Tract. A tract draining an abscess is termed a *sinus tract.* The sinus tract traverses from the deeper tissues to a lining or covering surface.

Fistula (Fistulous Tract). A fistulous tract is a tract connecting one lining surface to another lining surface.

Cellulitis. Cellulitis is a diffuse spreading necrotizing type of inflammation. A serous exudate is initially present but changes to a diffuse purulent exudate which spreads rapidly through the tissues.

Phlegmonous Inflammation (Phlegmon). When an infection spreads through musculature, the spreading inflammation may assume the form of a sheet confined by the fascial planes. This type of spreading inflammation is termed *phlegmonous inflammation.* The term *phlegmon* means an indurated part.

Gangrene and Gangrenous Inflammation. Gangrene may occur in any tissue. A subacute inflammatory process generally develops adjacent to the gangrene. *Noma* is an example of gangrenous inflammation.

Vincent's Angina. This angina is a painful acute fusospirochetal infection of the throat, oropharynx, palate and lymph nodes. Yellow-white ulcerations occur on the tonsillar fauces and halitosis is present.

Ludwig's Angina. Ludwig's Angina is a rapidly spreading gangrenous cellulitis originating in the submaxillary space. Extension of the angina occurs by continuity, involving the sublingual space. Ludwig's angina is characterized by a deep and tender swelling in the floor of the mouth involving submaxillary, sublingual and submental areas. The inflammation produces a hard wooden swelling in the floor of the mouth and neck causing an elevation of the tongue.

REGENERATION AND REPAIR OF TISSUES

Introduction to Regeneration and Repair of Tissues

Types of Repair. There are two basic types of repair. The first is a direct process of tissue repair by *restitution to integrity*. The second is an indirect process of repair by *substitution*. Restitution to integrity depends upon the type and the amount of exudate present in the affected tissue. The defect fills in by direct healing. In order for restitution to integrity to be accomplished, the tissue must first be capable of undergoing regeneration. *Resolution* is the disposal of debris in a healed inflammation. The phagocytic cells of the reticuloendothelial system are responsible for the disposal of the debris.

In the supporting tissues, fibroblasts regenerate and substitute for the lost cells whenever regeneration is impossible. In osseous tissue the osteoblast regenerates and replaces the lost osteocyte. The ductal epithelial cells of excretory ducts of salivary glands have the power of regeneration and are responsible for regeneration of acinar cells.

Substitution leads to a fibrous scar in the tissues. Connective tissue or osseous scar occurs wherever the basic architecture of the tissue is destroyed. Repair by substitution has three main components which are all of mesenchymal origin. Firstly, the proliferation of endothelial cells occurs as solid sheets and later as blood vessels. Secondly, a proliferation of fibroblasts takes place. Thirdly, blood borne and tissue borne cells emigrate into the involved area and a proliferation of these cells takes place.

Granulation tissue has a bright red color and a granular appearance. Granulation tissue supplies newly formed capillaries, contains fibroblasts and an infiltrate of lymphocytes, plasma cells and histiocytic cells. The main cells in chronic inflammation and granulation tissue associated with repair include lymphocytes, plasma cells, eosinophiles, monocytes and fibroblasts.

Repair by substitution in wounds is classified into healing by primary intention when the wound is closely approximated by sutures, and healing

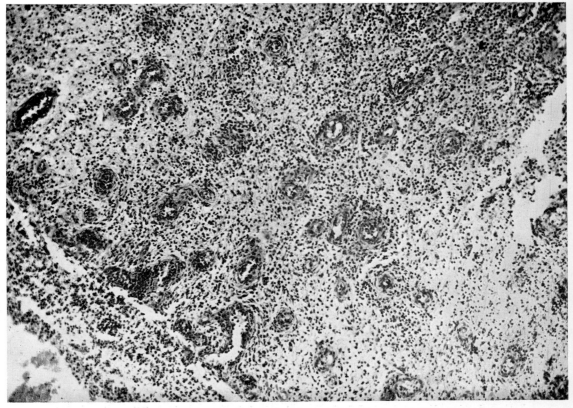

Figure 15. Granulation tissue. Notice the numerous capillaries, fibroblasts and chronic inflammatory cells which comprise granulation tissue.

by secondary intention when the edges of the wound are not approximated and thus repair must occur from the bottom of the wound upwards.

Essentials for Proper Wound Healing

A wound requires adequate nutrition supplied by means of an optimal blood supply. Adequate protein intake is vital since the elements of repair demand adequate amino acid nutrition. If vitamin C is absent, healing will be defective. Vitamin D, calcium and phosphorus are required in proper amounts for adequate repair of bone tissue. ACTH and cortisone decreases the amount of cellular proliferation during healing. During the first four days the tensile strength of a wound is unchanged. After the fourth or fifth day the tensile strength of the wound is progressively and rapidly increased and levels out at twelve to fourteen days. The strength of the wound indicates the degree of deposition of collagen fibers. The maximum strength of the wound is directly proportional to the deposition and intertwining of collagen fiber bundles.

Factors Preventing Healing

Failure of regeneration of the surface epithelium is generally due to a large wound. Scarring in the depths of the granulation tissue makes it more

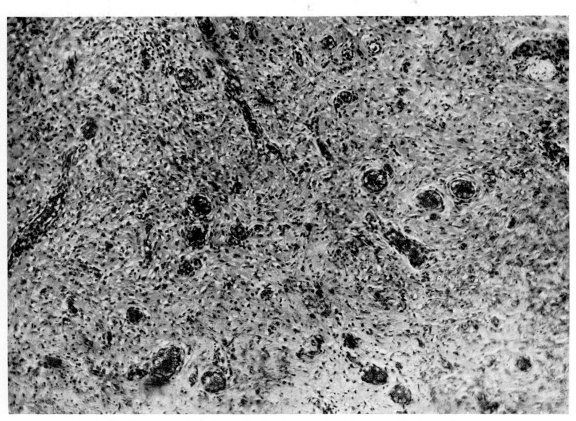

Figure 16. Healing wound, 3 days old. Notice the abundant capillaries and young fibroblasts. Collagen fibers have not formed at this early date.

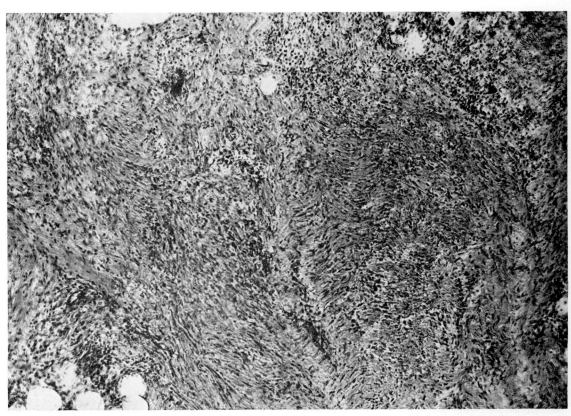

Figure 17. Healing wound, 19 days old. Notice the decrease in vascularity and abundance of collagen fibers and fibroblasts.

TABLE VI
FACTORS INFLUENCING WOUND HEALING

Essential to Healing	*Preventing Wound Healing*
High protein diet	Malnutrition (deficient amino
High vitamin C diet	acid and vitamin C)
Young age	Hypoalbumenemia
Minimal trauma or irritation	Senility
Minimal sutures	Chronic irritation
Slightly increased local	Freezing or chilling
temperature (warmth)	Toxemia (virulent infection)
No foreign body reaction	Virulent organisms in tissue
	Tight sutures
	Excessive trauma
	Foreign bodies
	Large defect or wide gap
	Prolonged ACTH or cortisone
	therapy
	Ionizing radiation

difficult for a wound to heal since scarring reduces the blood supply to the wound. Healing is delayed by failure of the exudate to be resolved, organized or lysed. Foreign bodies which remain in the inflammatory zone prevent healing.

CORRELATION OF PATHOLOGY WITH RESULTANT CLINICAL PROBLEMS

Healing of Bone Tissue

Differentiation of connective tissue cells is the preliminary process in the healing of bone fractures and extraction wounds. Following the fracture of a bone, the first mechanism is the formation of a hematoma. The hematoma becomes organized as fibroblasts proliferate into the mass of coagulated blood, fibrin, erythrocytes and serum. When connective tissue proliferates into the hematoma, capillaries and fibroblasts undergo mitotic division forming a young connective tissue. Undifferentiated mesenchymal cells migrate into the young connective tissue and fibroblasts differentiate into osteoblasts.

Classification of Fractures

A *traumatic fracture* occurs due to a momentary increase in force upon normal bone. A *pathologic fracture* is spontaneous and occurs under physiologic forces because the bone is involved by a pathologic process. In *incomplete fractures* the segments of bone remain approximated. In *complete fractures* both ends of the bone may remain approximated or become displaced.

Fractures may be classified as *open fractures,* if they communicate with the outer surface, or as *closed or simple fractures* if no communication exists with the outer surface. The basic mechanism of healing is similar in the closed and open fracture.

Healing of a Fracture of Long Bones

Following a fracture, the bone marrow is replaced by a hematoma. The hematoma is replaced by fibrous tissue forming a fibrous callus. In most areas of the fibrous callus, connective tissue forms directly into bone which is similar to developing membranous bone.

The callus may be subdivided into four divisions. The *anchoring callus* is the most peripheral and lateral cuff which attaches the callus to the free ends of the fractured long bone. A second callus develops between the two cuffs of the anchoring callus, the *bridging callus*. An area of the callus unites the ends of the fracture and is called the *uniting callus*. Bone formation closes the exposed marrow cavities. The latter is called the *sealing callus*. The transformation of the callus into bone tissue occurs in the connective tissue and takes place in all regions of the callus with the exception of the bridging callus. The bridging callus duplicates endochondral bone formation.

The bridging callus is composed of hyaline cartilage which undergoes calcification. Following calcification the cartilage is invaded by proliferating connective tissue cells. The calcified cartilage in the callus is resorbed by osteoclasts. After three to four weeks of healing, immature bone fills the entire defect created by the fracture. The filling in of mature bone occurs at approximately six months. Functional forces exerted upon the bone are responsible for remodelling. It may require years before remodelling is complete following the healing of a fracture. The healing process following the fracture of a long bone may be divided into the following six stages: the hematoma, fibrous callus, primary bony callus, secondary bony callus, reconstruction and apposition.

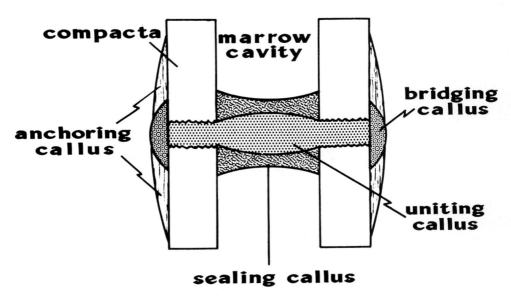

Figure 18. Diagrammatic representation of the healing of a fracture of a long bone showing the formation of the fibrous and cartilagenous callus (primary callus). The primary callus follows the organization of the hematoma. The bridging callus consists of cartilage. The uniting callus, anchoring callus, and sealing callus develop directly into bone.

Healing of a Jaw Fracture

The primary sequence of events in the healing of a fracture of the jaws is as follows: hemorrhage, blood clot, organization, granulation tissue and resolution. Fibroblasts and solid masses of endothelial cells migrate into the blood clot. The young granulation tissue that proliferates into the fracture site subsequently matures into fibrous connective tissue following resolution. Connective tissue unites the fractured ends of the jaw. The latter is in distinct contrast to the healing of a fracture of a long bone. Immature bone forms the initial bony callus of the fractured jaw. The fibrous connective tissue callus and immature bony callus extend beyond the limits of the jaw fracture. The excessive amount of immature bony callus must therefore be resorbed and replaced by mature lamellated bone. The terminal process is reconstruction of the mature bony callus according to the stresses placed upon the jaw.

Chapter 5

SPECIFIC GRANULOMATOUS INFLAMMATIONS

TUBERCULOSIS—A GRANULOMATOUS INFLAMMATORY
PROCESS CAUSED BY BACTERIA

Human Tuberculosis

Tuberculosis is a chronic granulomatous inflammatory process produced by the tubercle bacillus. Two species of tubercle bacilli are of importance in human pathology—*Mycotuberculosis hominis* (human) and the *Mycotuberculosis bovis* (bovine). Precisely how the tuberculous parasite acts in the host depends upon the number of tubercle bacilli at the portal of entry and the virulence of the organisms. The action of the host depends upon age, sex, race, previous exposure, i.e. immunization, constitution, nutritional status and the state of health.

Immunity and Sensitivity. Individuals who have never been previously exposed and become infected for the first time exhibit a different reaction to the tubercle bacillus than individuals who become reinfected. Immunity to tuberculosis is demonstrable as tissue immunity. The caseation necrosis within a tubercle represents a local tissue hypersensitivity response to the presence of the tubercle bacillus and a low immunity. The majority of infected individuals have an incomplete immunity; therefore, the tubercle bacilli grow after inoculation and spread to the regional lymph nodes. The primary lesion spreads to regional lymph nodes and both areas undergo caseation necrosis. When immunity is high, both the primary lesion and lymph node with caseation necrosis becomes encapsulated.

Primary Lesion of Tuberculosis. The primary lesion of tuberculosis consists of an infiltrate of monocytes, histiocytes and giant cells. A progressive accumulation of histiocytic cells forms tubercles wherever tubercle bacilli have proliferated. A *tubercle* is an avascular circumscribed structure surrounded by modified large round histiocytic cells. The histiocytic cells are termed *epithelioid histiocytes* because they appear similar to sheets of epithelium. Giant cells consisting of a large central zone of cytoplasm and multiple peripheral nuclei polarized toward the center are termed *Langhan's giant cells*.

The tubercle expands by coalescence with adjacent tubercles. As tissue immunity develops, the individual restricts the growth of organisms. The primary tubercle may occur on the hand with enlargement of the axillary lymph nodes. In human tuberculosis the lungs are generally the site of the primary lesion. The primary lesion in the lungs is termed the *Ghon tubercle*. A subpleural lesion is generally present in the lower part of the upper lobe and may spread to the pleura. The tracheobronchial lymph nodes readily become involved by the tubercular infection. A *Ghon complex* therefore develops.

Spread of Tuberculosis. Tubercle bacilli spread throughout the host (1) by an extension of the local infection to adjacent tissues, (2) by passing through existing body passages, (3) by lymphatic and hematogenous routes

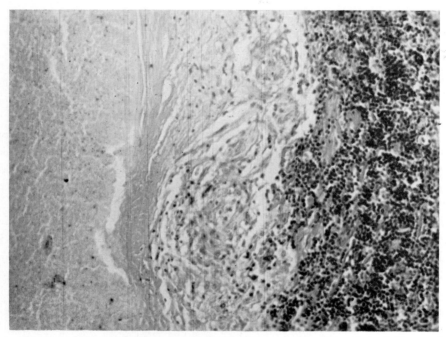

Figure 19. Tuberculosis of a lymph node. Notice the peripheral hyalinized fibrous tissue surrounding a central zone of caseation necrosis. The lesion eventually develops into a hyalinized fibrous nodule. The lymphoid and reticuloendothelial cells of the lymph node are evident at the periphery of the hyalinized fibrous tissue.

and (4) by implantation in body cavities. Organisms escape from the Ghon tubercle and generally spread by way of the lymphatics. If the primary site of infection is in the tonsil, the infection spreads to the cervical lymph nodes. An opaque, yellow caseous material is present in the faucial, pharyngeal or lingual tonsil when these areas are the portal of entry for the *Mycobacterium hominis*.

Miliary Tuberculosis. Miliary tuberculosis is due to the dissemination of tubercle bacilli either by extension from the lung or regional lymph node directly into a blood vessel or into the lymphatic vessels and subsequently into the blood stream. Multiple tubercles which develop in numerous organs are termed *miliary lesions*.

Specific Forms of Tuberculosis. *Scrofula* is tuberculosis involving the cervical chain of lymph nodes. It generally results from extension of primary tuberculosis of the tonsil through the lymphatics to the cervical lymph nodes. The clinician should be aware of this manifestation of tuberculosis when making a differential diagnosis of an enlargement in the neck.

Skin tuberculosis is termed *lupus vulgaris*. Tuberculosis may disseminate to the skin by way of the hematogenous route, or abrasions and cuts may be directly infected with tubercle bacilli.

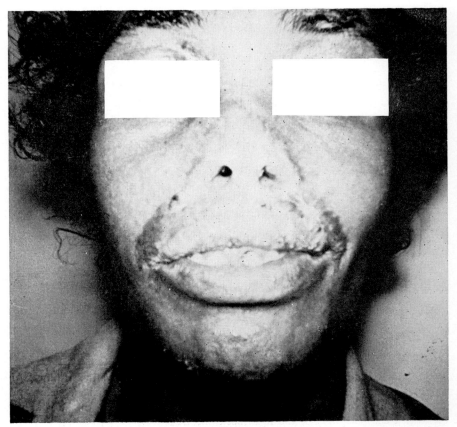

Figure 20. Lupus vulgaris of the lips and face (tuberculosis of the skin). Notice the localized form of tuberculosis of the skin. The epidermis is irregularly hypertrophic. Histopathologic changes in this case of lupus vulgaris include accumulations of epithelioid histiocytes, multinucleated giant cells and lymphocytes. No caseation necrosis is present.

Reinfection Tuberculosis. A special type of tuberculosis may develop following a healed Ghon complex termed *reinfection tuberculosis*. The reinfection phase of tuberculosis in adults involves the apical region of the lung. No lymph node lesions are present. The primary lesion may be apparent and the individual may have been immunized prior to the development of reinfection tuberculosis.

Liquefaction necrosis may develop in conglomerate caseous lesions. The enlarged area of liquefaction necrosis ruptures into a bronchus, producing the *cavitation of reinfection tuberculosis*. Coughing and expectoration of viable tubercle bacilli follows the development of cavitation. The expelled breath of a tuberculous patient due to coughing contains a fine spray which may contain numerous tubercle bacilli. The clinician and technician are likely to be exposed to the expelled breath of the tuberculous patient. Therefore, they should have a chest x-ray taken at least once a year.

Skin Test for Tuberculosis. In a tuberculin positive test the skin reaction consists of partial induration (wheal) and erythema. The tuberculin test indicates whether or not an individual has been previously infected with tubercle bacilli.

TABLE VII

GRANULOMATOUS INFLAMMATIONS ARE CHARACTERISTIC
OF THE FOLLOWING DISEASES

Tuberculosis	Schistosomiasis
Syphilis	Weber-Christian Disease (fat necrosis)
Sarcoidosis	Chagas disease
Leprosy	Fat necrosis
Granuloma inguinale	Brucellosis
Most fungal diseases (Coccidioidomycosis)	Tularemia
Beryllium pneumonitis	

TABLE VIII

PRIMARY AND REINFECTION TUBERCULOSIS IN THE GUINEA PIG

Type of Infection	Type of Animal	Inoculation at Local Site	Tissue Alteration at Site of Inoculation	Regional Lymph Nodes
Primary Lesion	Healthy guinea pig	Inoculate with tubercle bacillus	Slowly evolving progressive lesion. Lag occurs. Lesion appears in one week. Ulcerated lesion remains to death of guinea pig	Lymph nodes enlarged. Caseous necrosis
Super Infection (Reinfection)	Infected guinea pig	Inoculate with tubercle bacillus 2–3 weeks after initial infection	Area of induration develops rapidly. Ulceration and healing occurs before death of guinea pig	Lymph nodes not enlarged. Unaffected nodes. No caseation necrosis

TABLE IX

TUBERCULIN TESTS

Tuberculin negative	No skin sensitivity present to products of tubercle bacillus	Not previously exposed
Tuberculin positive	Skin reactivity after period of weeks	Previously exposed to primary infection

LEPROSY—AN INFECTIOUS GRANULOMA CAUSED BY BACTERIA

Leprosy (Hansen's disease) is caused by the acid fast bacillus, *Mycobacterium leprae*. Leprosy may be transmitted due to close contact. The disease is characterized by an extremely lengthy incubation period which ranges from five to twenty years. Leprosy has a chronic and protracted course. The

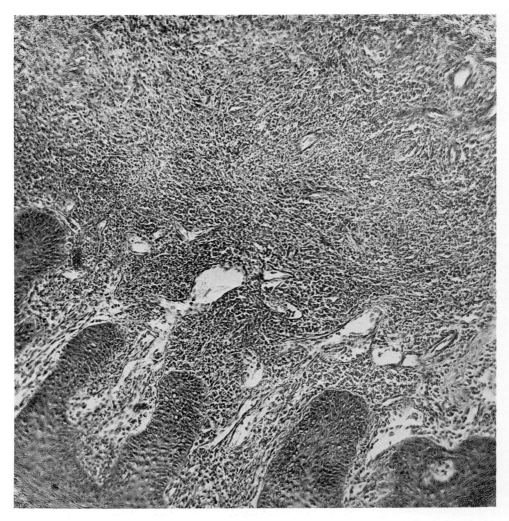

Figure 21. Leprosy involving the tongue. Notice the absence of the musculature of the tongue and its replacement by a peculiar granulomatous tissue reaction. The reaction is characterized by enlarged mononuclear cells with lipid in the cytoplasm producing the so-called foam cel's. The overlying epithelium is atrophic.

early lesions of leprosy occur as small macules in the skin. One type of macule contains numerous leprae bacilli, is *lepromin negative,* and is characteristic of *lepromatous leprosy.* A second type of macule contains few bacilli, is *lepromin positive,* and is characteristic of *tuberculoid leprosy.*

In the early phase of leprosy a cellular infiltration is present in the skin, and loss of hair occurs in a diffuse fashion. During the advanced phase of leprosy a massive cellular infiltrate takes place in the skin of the face producing a leonine face. The infected nasal mucosa may be scraped and the mucous membranes shown to contain numerous leprae bacilli.

Leprae bacilli within histiocytic cells and a cellular infiltrate are found in the peripheral nerves and myelinated nerve fibers. Ulcers which form in the skin generally impair sensation. Ulceration of the mucous membranes is a common finding during leprosy. No tissue necrosis develops during leprosy because of the low tissue sensitivity.

SYPHILIS—AN INFECTIOUS GRANULOMA CAUSED BY SPIROCHETAL ORGANISMS

Primary Syphilis. The primary site of inoculation of the *Treponema pallidum* occurs either in the genitals or in extra-genital tissues. An incubation period of three weeks is present before the primary lesion, the hard *chancre* develops at the site of the inoculation. The primary lesion is present for six weeks. It is a firm, indurated lesion which undergoes ulceration. The primary lesion contains a massive local infiltrate of lymphocytes, plasma cells and a proliferation of blood vessels. Lymphocytes and plasma cells are present in the walls of blood vessels. The endothelial cells of arteries and veins are swollen and the lumen is reduced in size.

Secondary Syphilis. The secondary lesions appear three to six weeks after the primary lesion and are widely distributed throughout the body. General lymphadenopathy is a common finding. The secondary lesions of syphilis are located in the skin producing macules and papules.

Tertiary Syphilis. Tertiary lesions occur from five to twenty years following the primary lesion. The tertiary lesion consists of a massive lymphocytic infiltrate and necrosis. Epithelioid cells, fibroblasts and Langhan's giant cells characterize the tertiary lesion. The necrosis and granulomatous response are termed *gummas*. The necrosis present in the gumma is termed *gummatous necrosis*. The tertiary lesion of syphilis occurs most frequently in the cardiovascular and central nervous systems.

Syphilis of the Central Nervous System. Tabes dorsalis is an example of meningovascular syphilis. This lesion occurs around the dorsal root of the spinal cord. Argyll Robertson pupils is a clinical manifestation of meningovascular syphilis. The pupils react in accommodation but do not react to light. Joint relaxation occurs and the patient with tabes dorsalis develops a sloppy gait.

Cardiovascular Syphilis. Syphilitic involvement of the blood vessels begins at the periphery of the vessel, advancing toward the lumen. Stenosis of the coronary arteries with coronary insufficiency, aortic insufficiency, saccular aneurysm, and myocardial involvement are the main cardiovascular findings.

Congenital Syphilis. Congenital syphilis occurs when the spirochetal organisms pass across the placenta after the eighteenth week of gestation. The infant develops skin lesions, rhinitis and tenderness over the long bones. Patients with congenital syphilis have frontal bossing, saber shins, interstitial keratitis and hydrarthrosis of the knee joint.

SARCOIDOSIS—AN INFECTIOUS GRANULOMA WITHOUT A PROVEN CAUSE

Sarcoidosis is a granulomatous disease of obscure etiology. The typical lesions are termed *hard tubercles* and are distributed in the lung, skin,

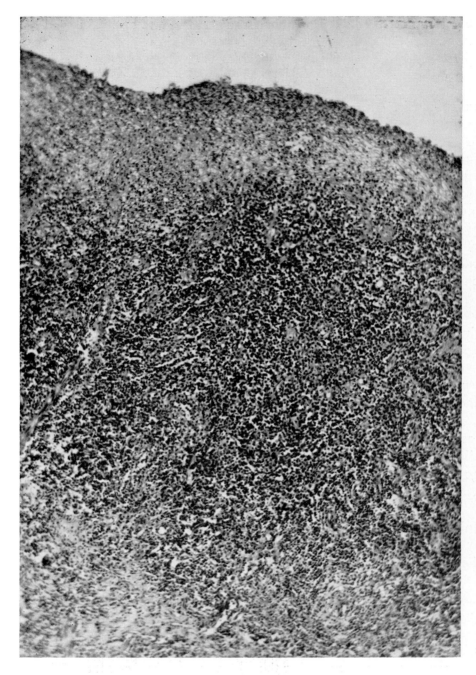

Figure 22. Chancre of the lip. Notice the ulceration of the covering epithelium, dense infiltrate of mononuclear cells (plasma cells, lymphocytes, histiocytes) in the lamina propria and increased number of capillaries. Spirochetes are very abundant in the chancre but are only demonstrable by special histochemical techniques.

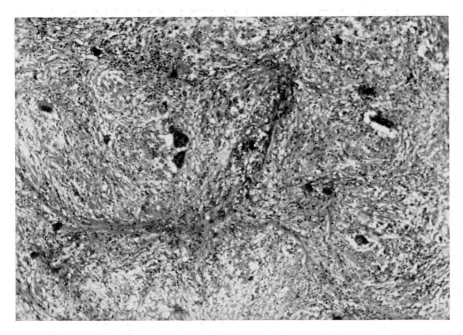

Figure 23. Boeck's sarcoidosis, a generalized systemic disease which may affect the heart. Notice the nodular or round accumulations of epithelioid histiocytic cells between atrophic cardiac muscle fibers. Caseation necrosis is not present and generally does not occur in the sarcoid lesion. Multinucleated giant cells are dispersed throughout the nodular arrangement of epithelioid cells.

lymph nodes, bones, liver, spleen, heart and skeletal muscle. The lesions of sarcoidosis consist of noncaseous granulomas. The sarcoid granuloma is discrete, well-circumscribed and surrounded by fibrous connective tissue. The giant cells of sarcoidosis may contain inclusion bodies termed *asteroids* and *Schaumann bodies*. Caseation necrosis is *not* present in sarcoidosis. The inclusion bodies should not be regarded as pathognomonic of sarcoidosis.

TULAREMIA—AN INFECTIOUS GRANULOMA CAUSED BY BACTERIA

Tularemia is a highly infectious granulomatous inflammation caused by *Pasteurella tularensis*. The organisms enter through the unbroken skin. In three to five days the primary site of inoculation develops a small elevated papular eruption. Indolent ulcers develop which require a prolonged period of healing.

TABLE X

IMMUNOLOGY, GROSS ANATOMIC, AND HISTOPATHOLOGIC FEATURES OF GRANULOMATOUS INFLAMMATIONS OF BACTERIAL ORIGIN

Granulomatous Inflammation of Bacterial Origin	Immunology	Gross Anatomic Features	Histopathologic Features
Tuberculosis	Ghon caseous stage—high immunity —high sensitivity Early Ghon tubercle—low immunity —low sensitivity Old Ghon tubercle—high immunity —low sensitivity Effect is due to bacterial bodies and soluble products, not to toxin.	Gross tubercle, firm, round, sharply demarcated, grey color Central necrosis occurs as a yellow mass Yellow central mass surrounded by grey rim of cells Consistency-firm to semifluid for central area Conglomerate tubercle—the outline is irregular, lobulated, diffuse The solitary tubercles are encapsulated, well defined, solid caseous centers with tiny satellites.	Tubercle has central mass of epithelioid cells surrounded by lymphocytes Central part is seat of necrosis Langhan's giant cells around periphery Primary complex-Ghon tubercle and nodes Necrosis of whole lesion
Syphilis	(1) Primary—chancre—low immunity —low sensitivity Duration—9 weeks	(1) Macule develops to indurated papule. Becomes eroded and a superficial ulcerated button-like lesion develops with adherent fibrin.	(1) Subepithelial tissues are densely infiltrated with lymphocytes, plasma cells and few macrophages. Capillary proliferation, slight fibroblastic activity. Few PMN leukocytes in ulceration. Perivascular infiltrate.
	(2) Secondary—mucous patches condylomata lata—low immunity keratotic papules—low sensitivity Duration—1–3 years	(2) A mucocutaneous eruption: macule, maculo-papular, papular, pustular, ulcerated. Focal superficial ulcers are mucous patches. Condylomata lata is flat warty growths on moist surfaces.	(2) Infiltration contains lymphocytes and plasma cells. Perivascular infiltration more evident. Macrophages, increased vascularity. Slight fibroblastic reaction. Hyperplasia of epithelium. Elongation of rete ridges. Endarteritis and endothelial proliferation. Intimal fibrosis in late secondary stage.
	(3) Tertiary—gumma—high immunity —high sensitivity Gumma has caseous center Duration—5–20 years	(3) Gumma is a focal nonsuppurating lesion with central necrosis.	(3) Caseous necrosis in center surrounded by proliferating vascular connective tissue. Infiltrated with lymphocytes, plasma cells, macrophages, Langhan's giant cells and epithelioid cells.

Leprosy—early phase (1) 　　　—indeterminate phase (2) 　　　—Lepro fever (3) Lepromatous leprosy Tuberculoid leprosy	Low sensitivity to lepra bacilli 5 to 20 year incubation period (1) Lepromin negative macule 　　Lepromatous leprosy 　　Low immunity 　　Low sensitivity (2) Lepromin positive 　　Tuberculoid type macule 　　Few bacilli 　　High immunity 　　Low sensitivity (3) Lepro fever 　　High immunity 　　Individual can destroy organisms	Macule—early lesion Hyperemia, erythema and hyperpigmentation or hypopigmentation Lesion contains lepro bacillus at terminal nerve radicles.	Acid fast bacilli in cells called Virchow cells Histiocytic cells with lipid and bacilli No caseous necrosis (noncaseous tubercle)

TABLE XI

IMMUNITY AND SENSITIVITY IN CHRONIC
GRANULOMATOUS INFLAMMATIONS

Disease	*Immunity*	*Sensitivity*
Chronic tuberculous osteomyelitis	high	high
Caseous bronchopneumonia	low	high
Ghon tubercle (early)	low	low
Miliary tuberculosis	low	high
Old ghon tubercle	high	low
Ghon tubercle (caseous stage)	high	high
Old or chronic tuberculosis	high	—
Caseous tuberculosis	—	high
Early or beginning tuberculosis	low	low
Proliferative obliterative endarteritis	high or intermediate	low
Primary syphilis (chancre)	low	low
Secondary syphilis (mucous patches, condylomata lata and keratotic papules)	low or high	low
Tertiary syphilis or gumma (focal lesions with central necrosis)	high	high
Latent periods of syphilis	low	low
Congenital syphilis	low	high
Mesaortitis (tertiary syphilis)	high	low
Syphilitic orchitis	high	low
Untreated syphilis	high	high
Inadequately treated syphilis (early)	low	low
Neurosyphilis	low	high
Meningovascular syphilis (early)	low	high
Paresis (early syphilis)	low	high
Tabes dorsalis (late syphilis)	low	high
Congenital syphilis (tertiary stage)	high	high
Lepromatous leprosy (negative lepromin)	low	low
Tuberculoid leprosy (positive lepromin)	high	low
Indeterminate leprosy (early-negative lepromin)	low	low
Glander's disease (late)	high	high
Bejel (positive Wasserman)	low	high
Granuloma inguinale	low	high
Lymphopathia venereum (late)	high	high
Tularemia (late stage-suppuration)	high	high
Yaws (early)	low	—
Yaws (late)	high	—
Brucellosis	low	high

Chapter 6

ACUTE INFECTIOUS DISEASES

PRINCIPLES OF INFECTIOUS DISEASES VERSUS INFLAMMATION

Definition of Infection. Infections are inflammations resulting from injury to tissues by living parasitic organisms.

Factors Related to Organisms. The lesion that develops in infectious diseases depends upon *pathogenicity, virulence,* mode of growth, products produced, adaptability, protective capsules, motility, tissue specificity and the number of organisms in the tissues.

Factors Related to the Tissues. Bacterial proteins are *necrotoxins* which are capable of destroying the tissues of the host. *Exotoxins* are secreted by the organisms. *Endotoxins* are liberated after death of the organisms. The *spreading factor* converts the hyaluronic acid gel of the tissues into a liquid. An *edema producing factor* is present in tissues. A *fibrinolysin factor* hastens the breakdown of fibrin in the exudate. *Coagulase* acts locally in tissues producing coagulation of plasma and fibrin formation. *Leukocidin* is present in infected tissues and is a poisonous compound to leukocytes. *Hemolysin* causes hemolysis of red blood cells in infected tissues.

Virulence and Adaptation of Living Agents of Disease. Bacteria are living agents capable of adaptations. The virulence of an organism is a mechanism of adaptation. A strain of organism may, through successive generations, pass on to their offspring an increase in virulence.

Bacterial Specificity. Some organisms grow poorly in one tissue but rapidly in another tissue.

Factors Related to the Host. *The constitution, age, nutrition, endocrine status, immunity and hypersensitivity, type of tissue involved* and *previous injury or disease* are the main factors. In diabetes mellitus the carbohydrate content of the tissues causes an increased susceptibility to infection. In vitamin A and vitamin C deficiencies, the tissues become more susceptible to infections. *Endocrines* influence the ability of tissues to resist infection. ACTH therapy acts to permit the spread of infections. Infections are common in hypoadrenalism, hypopituitarism and hypothyroidism. *Immunity* influences the invasion of organisms into the tissues. *Hypersensitivity* is an exaggerated antigen-antibody response producing widespread necrosis in tissue. *Previous injury or disease* influences the type of tissue reaction resulting from living organisms.

TABLE XII

SIGNIFICANT FACTORS RELATED TO THE ORGANISM
AND HOST IN INFECTIOUS DISEASES

Host—Parasite Relationship or Stress-Reaction Relationship

Factors Related to the Parasite	*Factors Related to the Host*
Toxicity (deleterious agent or action)	Immunity
Pathogenicity (ability of organism to produce pathologic change)	Nutrition
Virulence (varies in same organism and culture)	Endocrine Disorders
Presence of capsule	Previous trauma or injury
Size of organisms	Age
Rate of growth	Antibodies
Motility	Ability to produce phagocytic cells
Tissue specificity	Previous disease
Metabolism (varies in different hosts)	Ability of host to localize reaction

Organisms' Influence on Tissues. When living organisms produce necrosis of epithelial cells the resulting lesion is an *ulcer*. Organisms may cause necrosis and liquefaction of cells and the resulting lesion is an *abscess*. When bacterial toxins produce excessive tissue necrosis with putrefaction, the result is *gangrene*.

Systemic Effects of Infectious Diseases. The systemic effects of infectious diseases include chills, fever, malaise, nausea, vomiting, aching joints and loss of appetite.

Complications of Infectious Diseases. Complications are primarily due to the *spread of the infection* locally or systemically by way of the *vascular system*. The local spread of infection produces an abscess, cellulitis, sinus and *fistula*. The hematogenous spread of infection produces a bacteremia, septic thrombus, septicemia and pyemia. The diffuse spread of infection through the tissue produces a cellulitis.

Disturbances in Healing. *Failure of resolution* of an exudate results in a disturbance in healing. *Contraction* of collagenous tissue occurs during aging. Scar tissue pulls upon a joint with the development of a *contracture,* therefore the extremity cannot be extended.

Incidence of Bacteremia in Infections. Following a tonsillectomy, 30 percent of individuals develop a bacteremia. Mastication produces a transient bacteremia in 55 percent of individuals. After extraction of teeth, a *transient bacteremia* is present in 75 percent of individuals.

ACUTE BACTERIAL DISEASES

Staphylococcus Infections

Staphylococci are hemolytic organisms producing necrotoxins which are responsible for necrosis of epithelium, and enterotoxins which are responsible for food poisoning. Acute inflammatory lesions due to *Staphylococcus albus* drain spontaneously resulting in minimal necrosis. *Staphylococcus aureus* is more pathogenic than *Staphylococcus albus*. A *boil* or *furuncle* of the skin is due to *Staphylococcus aureus*. A *carbuncle* is a group of boils or a diffuse distribution of furuncles. Staphylococci produce *felons,* infected finger tips. When the staphylococcus infection occurs around the nail the infection is termed *paronychia*. Necrotoxins produced by staphylococci affect bone tissue by provoking necrosis and *osteomyelitis*. *Impetigo* is a staphylococcus infection of the epidermis of the skin. Superficial pustules develop but break down readily forming shallow ulcers. A staphylococcal bacteremia may result in *osteomyelitis* of bone tissue. Osteomyelitis due to *Staphylococcus aureus* is a chronic disease and is extremely difficult to eradicate.

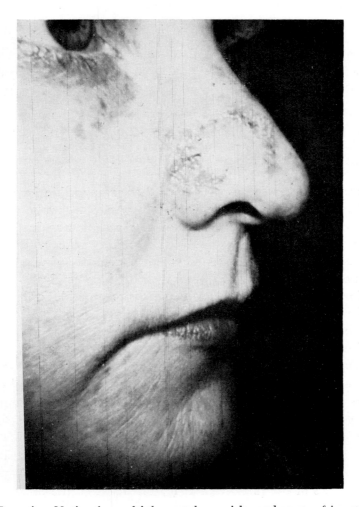

Figure 24. Impetigo. Notice the multiple pustules, vesicles and crusts of impetigo located on the nose, lower eyelid and face. The older lesions are encrusted and appear dark. The infection is caused by streptococci.

Streptococcal Infections

Streptococcus pyogenes or beta-hemolytic streptococci are the most pathogenic streptococci. Alpha- and gamma-hemolytic streptococci are the least pathogenic. Streptococcal organisms cause septicemia during wound infections of the hands and face.

Phlegmon, i.e. suppurative cellulitis is a spreading, diffuse, necrotizing and poorly outlined inflammation due to streptococcal organisms. *Erysipelas* is an acute group A hemolytic streptococcal inflammation involving the extracellular portion of the dermis. Erysipelas produces sharp well-defined borders in the affected tissues. The duration of the inflammation is from four days to two weeks. The inflammation is usually self-limited; however, septicemia is a possible complication. The *Quincy sore throat* and *retropharyngeal abscesses* are due to streptococcal infections. *Ludwig's angina* is a hemolytic streptococcal infection of the soft tissues of the neck, submandibular area, and floor of the mouth.

In *scarlet fever* a streptococcal septicemia is caused by beta-hemolytic streptococci. Pink skin rash, high fever, sore throat, involvement of the skin and mucous membranes and a *strawberry tongue* are the main symptoms. The mucous membranes and the skin frequently undergo ulceration.

Diplococcus Infections

Diplococcus pneumonia types 1, 2, and 3 are responsible for *lobar pneumonia*. Lobar pneumonia may be divided into red hepatization, gray hepatization and resolution. If failure of resolution occurs, carnification, abscess, or gangrene develops in the lung. When resolution takes place, the leukocytes liberate a fibrinolytic enzyme which produces a liquid exudate. Following failure of resolution the lung becomes solid, i.e. carnification is present.

Neisseria Gonorrhea. *Neisseria gonorrhea* is responsible for limited tissue necrosis. *Diplococcus gonococcus* provokes an acute suppurative infection of mucous membranes.

Neisseria Meningitdes. Exposure to *Neisseria meningococci* may result in *epidemic meningitis.* A bacteremia occurs in every case of meningococcus infection. Acute bacterial endocarditis may result from the bacteremia. A sore throat is the initial symptom; however, in twenty-four hours a septicemia is present. Multiple confluent petechial hemorrhages occur in the mucous membranes.

Pseudomonas Aeruginosa. Pseudomonas infections occur secondary to starvation, diabetes mellitus or following successful treatment with antibiotics. Cellulitis of the maxillofacial regions may be due to *Pseudomonas aeruginosa.*

Corynebacterium diphtheriae is the only pathogenic group of corynebacterium. Adults acquire immunity by contracting diphtheria or by immunization. Intoxication may occur with toxemia. The organisms remain on the surface of the pharynx and nasopharynx producing exotoxins which cause necrosis.

Hemophilus pertussis or *whooping cough* generally occurs in children under five years of age. A mild upper respiratory infection occurs accompanied by coughing. Severe coughing ensues which lasts from three to four weeks. Paroxysmal states of coughing occur every four to five hours.

Friedländer's bacillus occurs in debilitated individuals as a secondary infection causing a diffuse lobar or patchy type of pulmonary infection.

Typhoid Fever. Typhoid microorganisms enter the body through food or contaminated water and enter the lower gastrointestinal tract and Peyer's patches of the colon. As the disease progresses, lymphoid proliferation occurs in the reticuloendothelial system.

Ptomaine Poisoning. Food poisoning is generally due to *Staphylococcus aureus;* however, it may be due to *Clostridium botulinum.* When the organisms and toxins are ingested they are absorbed by the host and cause symptoms of ptomaine poisoning. Botulism is due to organisms which are capable of surviving for long periods of time. The organisms produce a potent neurotoxin.

Clostridium Tetani. *Clostridium tetani* grow within necrotic tissue. A true toxemia results along with a slight local reaction. The neurotoxin of Clostridium tetani is a stimulatory toxin producing clonic contraction of muscles of the jaws. The muscles of the face and mastication undergo contractures. The contractures are painful and spread rapidly to the trunk where every muscle undergoes contraction while the patient is conscious.

Clostridium Welchii. *Clostridium welchii* organisms are responsible for *gas gangrene.* Clostridium welchii grow in necrotic tissues producing an exotoxin that causes local necrosis of tissue due to the formation of gas.

Glanders Bacillus. Glanders bacillus penetrates intact skin, therefore, laboratory workers may develop glanders disease. Lymphadenopathy and septicemia develop with a generalized pustular rash.

Brucellosis. Brucellosis, also termed *undulant fever* is a viral disease characterized by nervous exhaustion, psychoneurosis, low-grade fever, weakness, malaise and joint pains.

Chapter 7

VIRAL, RICKETTSIAL AND FUNGAL DISEASES

VIRAL DISEASES

Introduction to Viral Diseases

Viruses are parasitic organisms which invade cells and utilize the metabolic systems of the cells to survive and reproduce. The virus may show an affinity for specific tissues. Neurotrophic viruses invade nervous tissue. Some cells are resistant to viruses and undergo proliferation while the viruses die. Other cells undergo degeneration and necrosis in the presence of viruses. Viruses multiply within cells forming colonies in the cytoplasm or nucleus. The viral colonies appear as homogeneous granules or small bodies termed *inclusion bodies.*

Antibodies may be produced following a viremia and are responsible for immunity. However, no immunity is produced when the viral organisms remain localized on the surface of cells. The common herpetic lesion of the lips is an example of a viral disease whereby the virus is localized on the surface of cells. No viremia develops following the herpes simplex infection; therefore, no immunity is present and the infection is recurrent as long as the virus remains in the cells. Dermatotrophic viruses, such as smallpox, affect the skin. The *Molluscum contagiosum* dermatotrophic virus causes a proliferation of epithelial cells.

Respiratory Viruses. Respiratory viruses affect the respiratory epithelium producing a transient viremia and an incomplete immunity. A number of strains of viruses actually localize in the upper respiratory tract during the *common cold.* Immunity is nonexistent following the common cold.

Influenza viruses affect respiratory membranes, small bronchi and the alveolar cells of the lung. *Atypical interstitial pneumonia* is due to a filterable respiratory virus which is accompanied by cold agglutinins in the blood of 60 percent of individuals.

Dermatotrophic Viruses. The dermatotrophic virus produces liquefaction necrosis and vesicle formation develops in the infected epithelium.

Smallpox virus produces areolar dermatotrophic lesions characterized by multiple macules in one generalized region. Scarring may result from the smallpox infection, producing a disfigured face.

Chickenpox is a mild dermatotrophic viral disease producing limited skin lesions. Permanent immunity to chickenpox results after the viral infection subsides. In children, herpes zoster virus produces chickenpox, and in the adult the same virus produces herpes zoster. Infection with either chickenpox or herpes zoster virus provides immunity against the other disease.

Herpes zoster virus affects the sensory nerves and sensory ganglia of the spinal cord and the nerve trunks of the skin of the face and abdomen. The herpes zoster virus affects sensory nerves causing a severe and disabling type of pain. Herpes zoster virus produces shingles on the skin. The lesions of herpes zoster may follow the course of the facial nerve.

Herpes simplex is a dermatotrophic viral infection producing vesicular lesions at the mucocutaneous junction of the lips and angle of the mouth. Infection does not produce an immunity to the herpes simplex virus. The virus lies dormant in the tissue; however, it may become activated.

Measles is a viral disease which produces a permanent immunity. The initial manifestations of measles appears in the oral mucosa and are termed *Koplik's spots*. Flattened lesions appear on the skin several days following the appearance of the Koplik's spots.

German measles or *rubella* is a mild viral disease which produces a small rash in the skin. When the viral disease occurs during pregnancy the virus may produce fetal abnormalities. The rubella virus passes through the placenta affecting all germ layers of the fetus.

Neurotrophic Viruses. Neurotrophic viruses invade the cells of the brain and spinal cord and ganglia. Rabies and poliomyelitis affect the ganglion cells.

Rabies is transmitted by dogs, wolves, cats and foxes by the inoculation of infected saliva under the skin. The relatively large rabies virus travels slowly along the route of nerves. Fortunately, the incubation period lasts from fifteen days to six months or one year. The maxillofacial region is a highly innervated anatomic region; therefore, a bite in this area is dangerous. Death will occur in ten days if the infected animal harbors the rabies virus in his brain and salivary glands. Chromatolysis of cells, destruction of cell nuclei and *negri bodies* are findings in the degenerated cytoplasm of affected cells. Negri inclusion bodies are the principle basis for the histopathologic diagnosis of rabies.

In man the prodromal symptoms of rabies are excitability, muscular twitch, hydrophobia, collapse and death. Fifteen injections of the rabies vaccine are required to produce an immunity in humans.

Poliomyelitis is due to a neurotrophic virus. Poliomyelitis virus enters the body through the nasal cavity, respiratory tract and intestinal mucosa. The virus travels along the axons of nerves and subsequently reaches the central nervous system. The virus is located in the anterior horns of the gray matter of the spinal cord, in the nuclei of the medulla oblongata, and in the motor area of the cortex. The virus stops suddenly when it passes the motor area of the cortex and enters the sensory areas of the brain.

The prodromal stage of poliomyelitis is characterized by muscular weak-

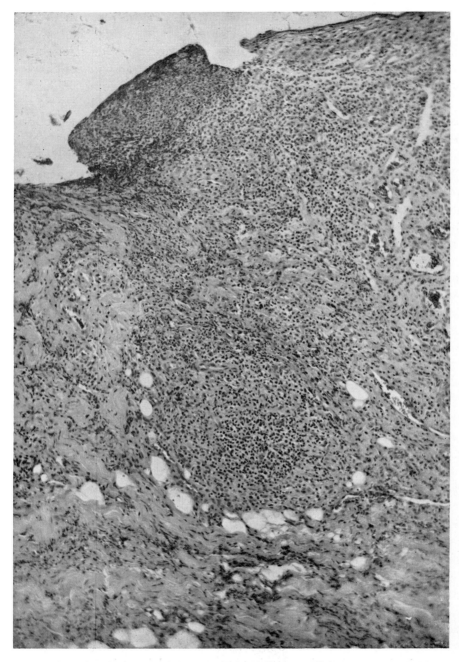

Figure 25. Herpes simplex. Notice the ulceration of the surface of this lesion. The bulla has ruptured and secondary infection is responsible for the presence of the inflammatory exudate and degenerated cells present in the connective tissue. The surface of the lesion is covered by an exudate composed of fibrin, polymorphonuclear leukocytes, necrotic tissue and debris.

ness and neck rigidity. When the lower neuron of the spinal cord is involved a flaccid paralysis results. When the spinal cord is affected above the lower neuron spastic paralysis results.

Miscellaneous Viral Infections. *Mumps* differs from the latter viral diseases because of the acute suppurative character of the exudate. *Infectious mononucleosis* is an acute infectious disease of unknown origin producing enlarged cervical lymph nodes. The disease produces atypical lymphocytes. The disease is characterized by oral and pharyngeal lesions. Laboratory findings include the following: leukocytosis (10,000 to 25,000), lymphocytosis (50 to 90 percent) and atypical lymphocytes. Heterophil antibodies are present in the circulating blood. *Yellow fever* is a viral disease transmitted by the mosquito. The disease produces necrosis of hepatic cells and periportal inflammation.

RICKETTSIAL DISEASES

Rickettsial organisms produce toxins and a proliferation of cells at the site of inoculation. A good immunity results following infection because of the presence of a rickettsemia and the production of antibodies.

Typhus Group. *Epidemic typhus* is due to *Rickettsia prowazekii*. The lumen of infected vessels may be blocked by Rickettsia prowazekii organisms. A cutaneous rash develops characterized by a poorly defined erythema of the skin. Hemorrhages occur in the skin. *Endemic typhus* is due to infection by *Rickettsia typhi*. This disease has a milder course than epidemic typhus.

Brill's disease is a mild form of epidemic typhus. A partial immunity follows the initial infection. *Epidemic hemorrhagic fever* follows a rapid clinical course with high fever, toxic and extensive hemorrhagic manifestations. Mucosal, skin, esophageal and gastric mucosal hemorrhages are present.

Spotted Fever Group (Ticks). *Rocky Mountain spotted fever* is due to infection by Rickettsia rickettsii. Hemorrhage is characteristic of Rocky Mountain spotted fever. Petechiae and ecchymosis are numerous on the skin and capsular surface of the kidney. *Boutonneuse fever* is a variety of spotted fever which occurs in the Mediterranean region.

Tsutsugamushi fever or *scrub typhus* is due to *Rickettsia tsutsugamushi*. The eschar lesion at the portal of entry is a crusted lesion. A small ulceration develops at the site of inoculation. Perivasculitis is present and a rash develops on the skin surface. *Q fever* is produced by *Rickettsia burneti* and is transmitted by ticks or by direct contact resulting in an interstitial pneumonitis and cyanosis.

Rickettsial pox is a self-limiting, acute febrile disease caused by *Rickettsia akari*. Rickettsial pox is characterized by an initial lesion at the site of infection, fever persisting for approximately one week and a papulovesicular rash. The lesions of rickettsial pox are discrete, abundant or scanty in distribution. Papules and vesicles are observed on the skin and tongue.

PROTOZOAL INFECTIONS

Leishmaniasis. Leishmaniasis is caused by *Leishmania donovani* which produces a recurrent fever, anemia and leukocytopenia. The clinical manifestations of leishmaniasis are chronic ulcers with sharply demarcated borders. Secondary infection is common.

FUNGAL DISEASES

Deep Fungi

Actinomycosis is produced by *Actinomycosis bovis* and *Actinomycosis israeli*. In the head and neck region actinomycosis produces a cervical or facial chronic granulomatous inflammation. Sixty percent of the fungi gain entrance into the body through the oral tissues, tonsillar crypts or pharynx. Chronic drainage follows the development of sinus tracts which prolongs the healing of lesions. The diagnosis of actinomycosis depends upon finding the actinomycotic organism in the infected tissue. Drainage of pus occurs from the lesions of actinomycosis. The pus contains tiny yellow sulfur granules in a tangled mass. Actinomycosis of the jaw is termed *lumpy jaw*.

North American blastomycosis produces warty elevated ulcerations in the cutaneous tissue of the lips, upper face, back and neck. Secondary blastomycosis is a systemic fungal disease which may involve any tissue. Blastomycotic organisms are disseminated by way of the blood stream. *South American blastomycosis* produces a swelling of the neck due to infected cervical lymph nodes. The organisms enter the body through the skin and mucous membrane.

Cryptococcosis (torula) is a fungal disease which produces a fatal pulmonary infection. The fungi enter the body through the respiratory and intestinal tracts.

Histoplasmosis is an airborne fungal infection involving infants and children. The histoplasmosis fungi live within macrophages throughout the body and produce a granulomatous reaction.

Coccidioidomycosis is a fungal disease primarily occurring in the San Joaquin Valley and southwestern region of the United States. The fungi enter the body by inhalation of contaminated dust. Coccidioidomycotic chronic pulmonary lesions undergo cavitation, necrosis, and abscess formation.

Sporotrichosis is a rare fungal infection in humans. The portal of entry is through the skin and mucous membrane. Local manifestations occur at the site of invasion after a three to four week incubation period. A sporo-

Figure 26 A and B. Actinomycosis of the parotid gland. Notice the organisms growing in the parotid gland in colonies consisting of a mass of filaments surrounded by projections, i.e. clubs. The ray fungus is surrounded by an abscess. Numerous leukocytes are present in the area of suppuration. Mononuclear cells and granulation tissue surround the abscess.   →

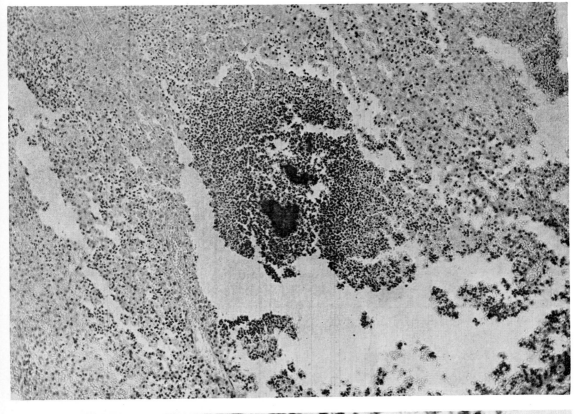

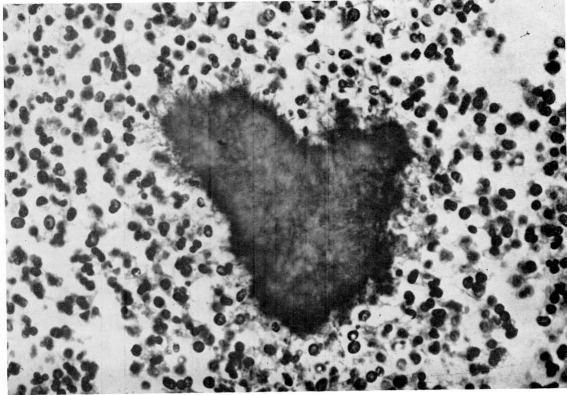

trichotic chancre is an ulcerated red papule discharging a thin watery fluid at the site of invasion.

Superficial Fungi

Candidiasis or *moniliasis* is a superficial infection due to *Candida albicans*. *Candida albicans* is common in the mucous membranes during the early and terminal years of life. Systemic and topical antibiotic therapy upsets the normal balance of bacteria and fungi. Fungi exert an inhibitory effect on the growth of bacteria. Although antibiotics destroy certain strains of bacteria, *Candida albicans* proliferates and becomes the predominant flora on mucous membrane.

Aspergillosis is due to aspergillus, a weak fungal invader that grows on mucous membranes. Aspergillus produces an infection in the gastrointestinal tract as a complication of prolonged antibiotic therapy. *Ringworm* is caused by a filamentous fungus which grows in the keratin layer of the skin and skin appendages. Blisters, ulcerations, and cracking of the skin develop as a result of ringworm infection.

Chapter 8

DISTURBANCES IN GROWTH AND DIFFERENTIATION AND NEOPLASIA

DISTURBANCES IN THE GROWTH OF CELLS

Cell Metamorphosis

Atrophy is an acquired reduction in the size of the units of a tissue which has attained the adult functioning size. Atrophy of the intercellular tissue indicates that a reduction is present in the amount of tissue forming cartilage, bone and ligaments. Atrophy results following infection with the poliomyelitis virus. Atrophy of muscles occurs in rheumatoid arthritis. In atrophic parotid glands, fatty ingrowth may produce a normal clinical picture.

In cellular atrophy the reduction occurs at the expense of the cytoplasm of cells. Malnutrition, inanition, abnormal pressure, and irradiation are some of the factors responsible for initiating atrophy of cells. During starvation an extreme degree of generalized atrophy takes place. Local atrophy of tissues is due to impairment of vessel walls. Atrophy of tissues may be induced by excessive pressure. When excessive pressure is present, the blood supply to the tissue is reduced resulting in atrophy and the production of an ulcer. In organs with ductal excretory systems an obstruction of the ductal system causes an increase in pressure, resulting in atrophy. In salivary glands an obstruction causes dilatation of the major excretory ducts resulting in atrophy.

The atrophy which accompanies aging of tissues is due to a reduction in the caliber of arteries. Atrophy is a reversible change in cells. However, atrophy may remain as a permanent state or lead to the death of cells.

Hypertrophy is an acquired increase in the size of tissues due to an increase in the size of individual cells comprising the tissue. *Compensatory hypertrophy* is an acquired increase in the size of an organ due to the loss of one member of a paired organ system. The individual cells in the remaining organ undergo an increase in size. Hypertrophy of the skin and mucous membranes is an increase in the size of cells associated with increased function or frictional forces. Hyperplasia is more common than hypertrophy in the mucous membranes. *Muscular hypertrophy* is an increase in the size of muscle cells due to increased functional demands. *Dystrophy* refers to alterations due to a lack of nutrition and is associated with additional factors. During dystrophy of muscles there is a decrease in the size of muscle cells in addition to necrosis of cells.

Agenesis, Plasia, Aplasia, Hypoplasia, Hyperplasia and Metaplasia of Cells

Agenesis indicates that a tissue was never formed. *Plasia* is multiplication of individual units. *Aplasia* is the minimal development of a tissue lacking complete maturation and development to an adult functioning unit. *Hypoplasia* is present where there has been inadequate proliferation of cells, but greater proliferation than minimal development of the tissue. The tissue is reduced in size during hypoplasia. *Hyperplasia* is an excessive multiplication of component cells. Reactive hyperplasia occurs in callus formation during the healing of a fracture. Hyperplasia occurs in the skin and mucous membranes. Hyperplasia may occur in the keratinized layer of the skin. The latter represents physiologic hyperplasia. Hyperplasia may take place in the basal cell layer of the epithelium of the skin and mucous membranes and represents pathologic hyperplasia.

The *keloid* is hyperplasia of the connective tissue of the corium of the skin. The keloid is seen more often in Negroes than Caucasians. It appears to be due to an injury whereby the healing process is excessive in character. The keloid may be classified between hyperplasia and neoplasia.

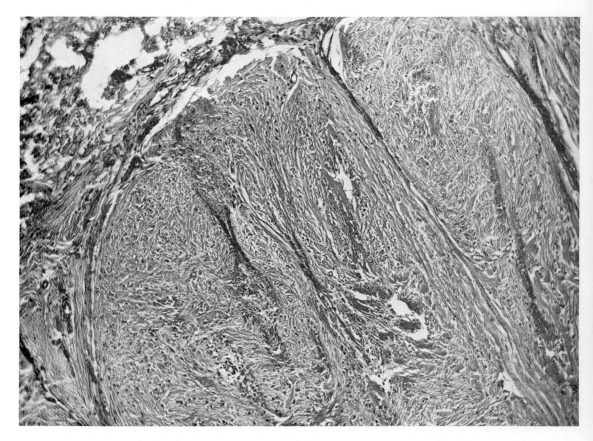

Figure 27. Keloid of the skin. Notice the bundles of mature and dense fibrous connective tissue in the submucosa of the skin. Mitoses are uncommon and skin appendages are absent.

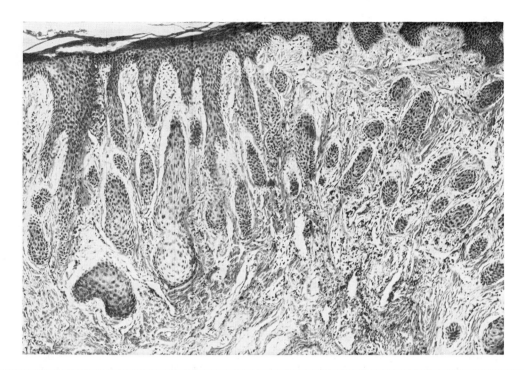

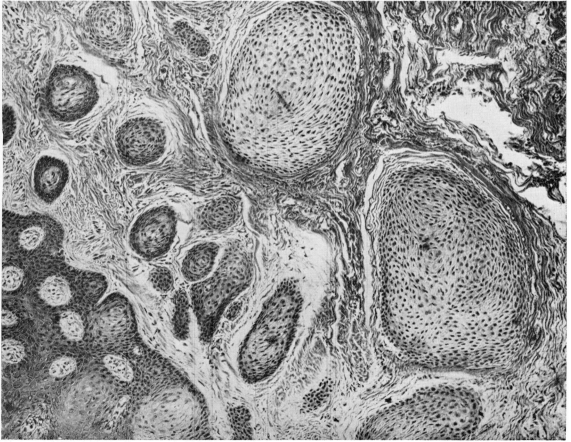

Figure 28 A and B. Pseudoepitheliomatous hyperplasia. Notice that the epithelial hyperplasia appears similar to a squamous cell carcinoma. There is an absence of dyskeratosis, the cells are more regular and are confined by an intact basement membrane.

Hyperplasia of the skin and mucous membranes is common. A great increase occurs in the hornified layer which clinically causes the mucous membranes to become white (hyperkeratosis). Hyperplasia of the mucous membranes and skin is the result of an increase in the number of cells. Hyperplasia is an enlargement of tissues associated with inflammation, endocrine disturbances and pharmacologic agents. Hypertrophy and hyperplasia of the mucous membranes and skin may occur simultaneously so that an increase in the number of cells also indicates an increase in the size of cells. Hyperplasia of ductal epithelium may take place in the excretory ducts of salivary glands. Squamous metaplasia and proliferation of ductal epithelium may be present in excretory ducts. Mucous glands have dilated excretory ducts during hyperplasia. The latter ducts undergo papillomatous hyperplasia and/or squamous metaplasia of ductal epithelium.

Hyperplasia is a common occurrence in the mucous membranes. The redundant hyperplastic tissue may be due to an irritation. Breast hyperplasia is produced by hormonal imbalance, such as excessive estrogenic hormone. The latter cells are governed by estrogenic hormones. *Pseudo-epitheliomatous hyperplasia* is a form of epithelial hyperplasia which may appear histologically similar to the squamous cell carcinoma. However, the epithelium ceases to proliferate. The epithelium is well differentiated and fails to demonstrate dyskeratosis.

Metaplasia of cells is a process whereby one cell type is transformed into another cell type. The transformation involves a change in the form and function of the metaplastic cell. Metaplasia occurs in the excetory ducts of salivary glands transforming the columnar cells into squamous cells. The degenerated columnar cells are replaced by squamous cells which originate from the undifferentiated reserve cell layer. During vitamin A deficiency the salivary gland ducts undergo metaplasia of their epithelial lining cells to keratinized squamous epithelium. Osseous metaplasia of muscle tissue may follow trauma. Metaplasia occurs in connective tissue cells with a transformation into cartilage or bone. Chondromatous metaplasia may occur in the mucous membranes following chronic irritation.

INTRODUCTION TO NEOPLASIA

Definitions

Tumor is a symptom of a disease, i.e. a swelling associated with inflammation, neoplasia, and hyperplasia. *Hamartoma* is an overexpression of tissue which serves no useful function. Hamartomas consist of normal constituents of the region arranged in an abnormal manner. *Choristoma* is an overdevelopment of tissue not normally present in the particular tissue. The latter overgrowth of tissue is derived from displaced anlagen.

Neoplasia refers to a specific pathologic process occurring in tissues and organs of the body. Neoplasia refers to a pathologic process whereby cells proliferate above and beyond the normal. Neoplasia is *one* process of unrestricted growth showing aggressiveness, invasion and metastases. The neoplastic process passes through several stages. The first stage is the conditioning of tissue resulting in dormant cells with neoplastic potential. In the triggering stage the dormant cells are activated to proliferating neoplastic cells. The final stage includes expansion, infiltration and metastases of the growing neoplasm. *Malignant* refers to a clinical behavior pattern elicited by a neoplasm. *Benign* describes the clinical behavior pattern of a neoplasm.

ETIOLOGY OF NEOPLASIA

While the precise etiology of neoplasia is obscure, extrinsic and intrinsic contributing factors are present.

Extrinsic Factors

In regions where the maximum amount of extrinsic *actinic radiation* occurs, one finds the highest prevalence of lip and skin neoplasms. Chromium and silica dusts are associated with the production of pulmonary carcinoma (cancer). Workers in the radium dial industry develop neoplasms of the bone marrow. The application of x-rays, coal tar and coal tar derivatives, tobacco and aniline dyes contribute to the development of neoplasia. Pipe smoking is a contributing factor to carcinoma of the lower lip. Aniline dyes are contributing factors to the development of neoplasms of the bladder. Benzene inhaled as fumes is a contributing factor to leukemia. Excessive smoking is a contributing factor to carcinoma of the lung. Tars, oils, petroleum, oily smegma, chutta (cigar) and khangri (charcoal) are exogenous carcinogens. Inorganic arsenic is carcinogenic to humans. Coal tar pitch is carcinogenic. Hot cutting oils may produce skin (epidermal) neoplasm. Carcinoma may occur in regions of a burn scar, in thermal and chemical burns, roentgen-ray dermatoses, chronic osteomyelitis, chronic sinuses and in tar and oil dermatoses. Butter yellow dye produces carcinoma of the liver in rats. Pellets of pyrene cause neoplasia at the site of chemical irritation. Radioactive strontium stored in bone tissue and radioactive gold stored in the bone marrow represent contributing factors to neoplasms of bone. *Viruses* have been implicated as an etiologic agent in human neoplasms. At the present time, the viral theory of neoplasia has gained considerable prominence.

Intrinsic Factors

Heredity or chromosomal defects are intrinsic contributing factors to the development of neoplasms. A high incidence of neoplasia is found in some families. Endocrine disorders and hormonal influences represent intrinsic contributing factors. Age, sex, race, genetic constitution, and alterations in cellular metabolism influence the production of neoplasia. All of the etiologic factors that act selectively on tissues act by repetitive injury and their effect is accumulative.

Chronic Irritation and Neoplasia. Chronic irritation may play a contributory role in the production of some neoplasms. The latter irritation factor must represent a specific type of irritation, occurring under very specific conditions. Individuals who have had osteomyelitis of bone tissue for a period of forty to fifty years with multiple sinuses may develop carcinoma at the exit of a draining sinus.

EPITHELIAL NEOPLASMS

The benign epithelial neoplasms utilize the growth form of the neoplasm as the prefix and add the suffix "oma." Malignant epithelial neoplasms are termed *carcinomas*. The *adenoma* is a benign glandular neoplasm of epithelial origin. The *adenocarcinoma* is a malignant glandular neoplasm of epithelial origin.

MESENCHYMAL NEOPLASMS

The *lipoma* is a benign neoplasm of fat tissue and the *fibroma* is a benign neoplasm of fibrous connective tissue. Malignant neoplasms of mesenchymal origin are termed *sarcomas*.

CHARACTERISTICS OF MALIGNANT NEOPLASMS

Malignant neoplasms grow with unlimited invasion of the adjacent tissue. Malignant neoplasms generally show a rapid rate of growth. The number of chromosomes in neoplastic cells may be double or triple the normal number. Nuclear and cellular pleomorphism are prominent features of malignant cells. Neoplastic cells show low differentiation, bizarre forms, loss of polarity and anaplasia. The failure of cells to differentiate is termed *anaplasia*. The more anaplastic the neoplasm, the less differentiated the cells

TABLE XIII-A
CRITERION OF MALIGNANCY IN CARCINOMA

Pleomorphism	Invasiveness
Hyperchromatism	Very cellular
Dyskeratosis	The deeper the neoplasm the
Abnormal mitosis	worse the prognosis
Anaplasia	Cellular irregularity
Site	Atypism

TABLE XIII-B
CLINICAL BEHAVIOR OF BENIGN AND MALIGNANT NEOPLASMS

Benign (Innocent)	*Malignant*
Grows by expansion	Grows by infiltration
Grows slowly	High mitotic activity
Compresses neighboring tissue (tissue atrophy)	Cells produce metastases
	Routes of invasion include intercellular pathways and vessel embolism
Interferes with blood supply (pressure resorption)	Primary route of carcinoma is through lymphatics, secondary route through blood vessels
Encapsulated	
Fills lumen of glands due to dilatation of wall by neoplasm	In sarcomas primary route is through blood vessels

TABLE XIII-C

SENSITIVITY OF TISSUES TO IRRADIATION

1. Lymphoid tissue and bone marrow	*most sensitive*
2. Epithelial cells, and salivary gland	
3. Endothelium of vessels	
4. Connective tissue	
5. Muscle, bone and nerves	*least sensitive*

comprising the neoplasm and the more malignant is the clinical behavior pattern. Malignant neoplasms have a tendency to recur after removal and following irradiation.

Malignant neoplasms spread to distant organs producing metastatic neoplasms. Every malignant neoplasm does not produce metastatic lesions. Carcinoma *in situ* does not metastasize. Basal cell carcinomas of the lip or skin do not metastasize.

SPREAD OF MALIGNANT NEOPLASMS

Malignant neoplasms spread by invading the surrounding tissues. Malignant cells may be transported mechanically, following separation from the main neoplastic mass, to the gastrointestinal or respiratory tracts. Malignant neoplasms spread by permeation through the lymphatics. The embolic spread of neoplastic cells is the primary manner of transportation through the lymphatics. Malignant neoplasms may spread by invading the blood vessels. Metastases from neoplasms occur by way of veins to the lungs, the portal circulation to the liver, and the lymphatics to the regional lymph nodes.

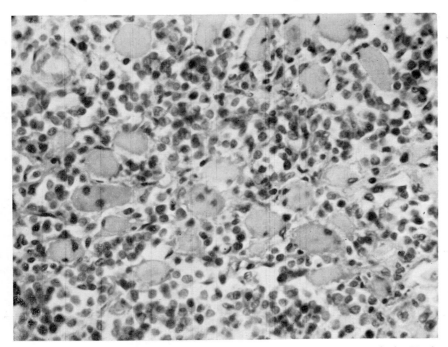

Figure 29. Invasion and destruction of skeletal muscle by malignant neoplasia. Notice the spread of cells of this neoplasm by direct invasion of the adjacent skeletal muscle. The numerous neoplastic cells are surrounding the atrophic and degenerating muscle cells.

CHARACTERISTICS OF BENIGN NEOPLASMS

Benign neoplasms grow by expansion and are generally encapsulated by fibrous connective tissue. Some benign neoplasms show an absence of a connective tissue capsule. A few benign neoplasms locally infiltrate the immediate surrounding tisue. A few benign neoplasms may undergo malignant transformation. Benign neoplasms grow slowly, are self-limiting, and may become arrested in their growth.

REACTION OF BONE TISSUE TO NEOPLASMS

Regardless of the type of primary or metastatic neoplasm, the reaction of bone tissue is always similar. The primary reaction is characterized by resorption of bone due to pressure from proliferating neoplastic cells. The secondary reaction is characterized by apposition of new bone.

CLINICAL DIAGNOSIS OF BENIGN AND MALIGNANT NEOPLASMS

Clinically and roentgenographically, it is difficult to differentiate, with certainty, the benign from the malignant neoplasm. Therefore, all neoplasms should be biopsied and submitted for histopathologic examination. When the lesion is small, it is good judgment to surgically excise it in its entirety (excisional biopsy) . When the lesion is large it is good judgment to do a preliminary incisional biopsy. Biopsy of a neoplasm does not force neoplastic cells into the lymphatics and therefore does not speed metastases.

TREATMENT OF NEOPLASIA

The treatment of malignant neoplasms includes surgery, external irradiation, surface radium, interstitial radiation, radium needle implants, radioisotopes and chemotherapeutic agents. The sensitivity of neoplasms to irradiation depends upon the degree of differentiation of the neoplasm. The more differentiated the neoplastic tissue, the more resistant it becomes to irradiation.

IRRADIATION AND OSTEORADIONECROSIS OF BONE

Irradiation therapy for neoplasms may result in osteoradionecrosis of bone tissue. When the dentition is present in individuals requiring irradiation therapy, preirradiation extractions become a *vital and imperative* matter. The removal of teeth in the path of the irradiation prior to therapy decreases the incidence of postradiation necrosis of the jaws. The opportunities for osteoradionecrosis are decidedly reduced when an intact mucous mucosa is present.

METASTATIC NEOPLASMS TO BONE TISSUE FROM DISTANT PRIMARY SITES

The primary neoplasms most frequently metastasizing to bone tissue result from carcinomas of the breast, thyroid, lung, kidney, testes, uterus, and

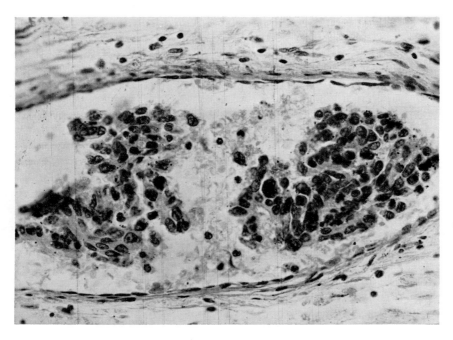

Figure 30. Tumor cell embolism. Notice the neoplastic cells of an adenocarcinoma invading the lumen of a blood vessel. Some of the neoplastic cells show karyorrhexis, pyknosis and karyolysis.

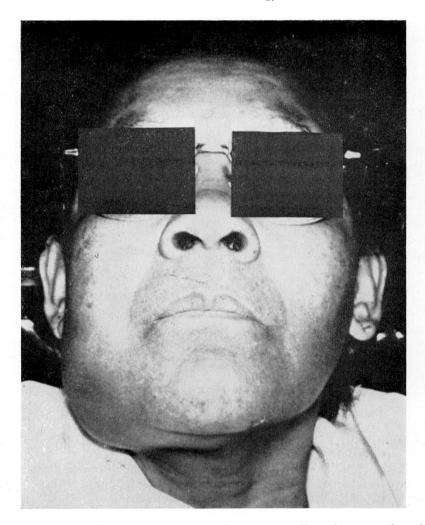

Figure 31. Metastases from a primary intraoral squamous cell carcinoma to the submandibular lymph nodes. Notice the lymphadenopathy involving the posterior and middle submaxillary lymph nodes.

sigmoid colon. The symptoms most commonly noted are pain, swelling, tenderness, paresthesia, numbness and neoplastic tissue at the site of metastases.

PATHOLOGY OF INDIVIDUAL NEOPLASMS

Benign Neoplasms of Epithelial Origin

The *papilloma* is a benign epithelial neoplasm which arises from the stratified squamous epithelium of the mucous membrane. The papilloma consists of projections of squamous epithelium supported by a thin core of connective tissue carrying blood vessels. The *adenoma* occurs in the glandular structures of the body. The multiplication of glandular elements forms an encapsulated adenoma.

The epithelial cells forming the glandular elements are capable of secreting a fluid leading to distention of the glandular spaces and development of the *cystadenoma* and the *papillary cystadenoma* of the salivary glands. The *pleomorphic adenoma* is a benign neoplasm of the salivary glands. Seventy-five percent of all salivary gland neoplasms are pleomorphic adenomas. The pleomorphic adenoma grows slowly. When the adenoma undergoes malignant transformation it grows rapidly and causes ulceration of the overlying surface. Histopathologically, the neoplasm is composed of basophilic epithelial cells which form ducts, acini, chords and nests.

Malignant Neoplasms of Epithelial Origin

Carcinoma is the most common malignant epithelial neoplasm of the skin and mucous membrane. There are several histologic types of carcinomas— squamous cell carcinoma, basal cell carcinoma and adenocarcinoma. The squamous cell carcinoma occurs on the lower and upper lips, oral mucosa, larynx, pharynx, large bronchi, esophagus and skin. The adenocarcinoma arises from the salivary glands.

The squamous cell carcinoma may be preceded by a thickened and dyskeratotic epithelium. Carcinoma may proliferate in the following gross forms: papillary (exophytic) growth, endophytic bulky mass, and ulcerated (infiltrating) growth. In the infiltrating carcinoma the margins of the neoplasm are indistinct. Carcinoma cells infiltrate the surrounding tissue spaces, invade the lymphatic channels and grow along the perineural lymphatics. Tumor cell emboli form in the lymphatics and are carried to regional and distant lymph nodes. Regional lymph node enlargement generally accompanies the carcinoma.

Squamous cell carcinoma occurs in deep fissures, furrows, or thickened epithelium (mucous membrane and skin). If the diagnosis of carcinoma is made when the neoplasm is less than 2 mm in diameter, a relatively good prognosis exists. The epidermoid carcinoma may be extremely difficult to diagnose clinically. The epidermoid carcinoma may appear clinically as an ulcer with an indurated border. Histologically, the epidermoid carcinoma is composed of irregular masses of squamous epithelium which infiltrates the lamina propria, submucosa, muscle and bone tissue. The keratin pearls are characteristic of a well-differentiated squamous cell carcinoma. In the undifferentiated squamous cell carcinoma the cells are characterized by great variation in size and shape and in staining characteristics.

Grading of squamous cell carcinoma indicates the degree of malignancy of the neoplasm. The epidermoid carcinoma may be divided into four grades depending upon the loss of differentiation, the degree of hyperchromatism and the number and abnormality of mitotic figures. Grade 1 is the most differentiated squamous cell carcinoma and therefore the least malignant of the four grades. Grade 1 consists of 75 percent or more of differentiated cells and 25 percent of undifferentiated cells. Grade 2 consists of 50 percent differentiated cells and 50 percent immature cells. Grade 3 consists of 25

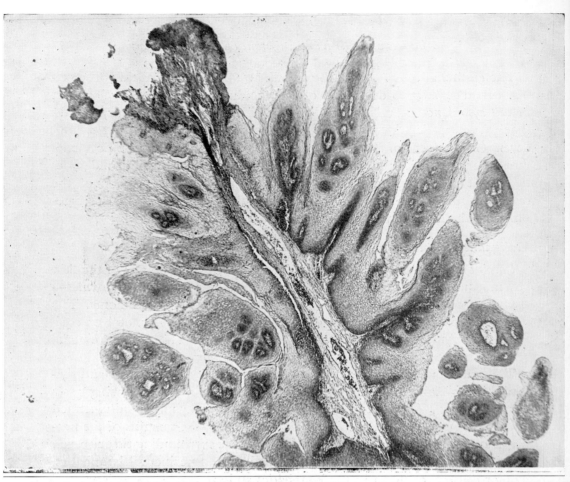

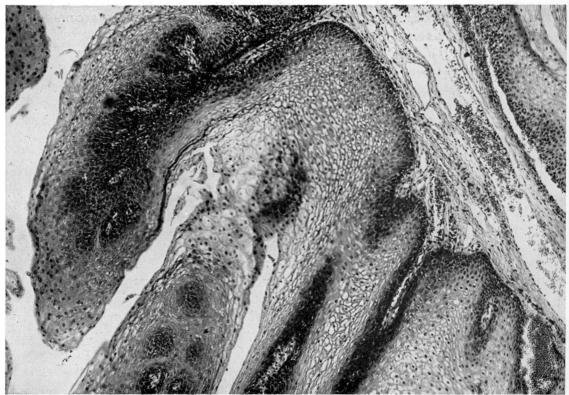

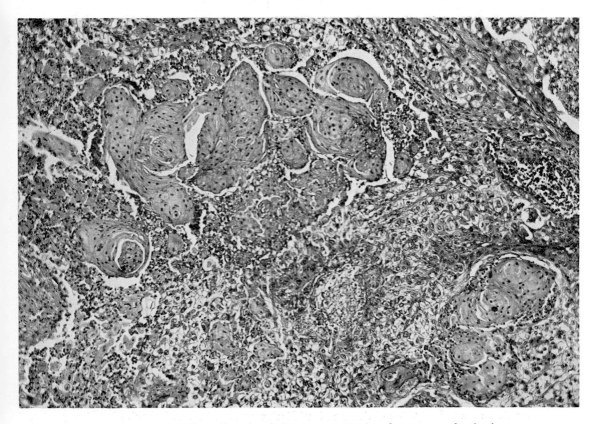

Figure 33. Squamous cell carcinoma of the tongue. Notice the masses of cohesive squamous epithelial cells replacing the musculature of the tongue. No normal tissue is present in this section. The squamous cells contain hyperchromatic nuclei and vary in size and shape. Chronic inflammatory cells infiltrate the small amount of connective tissue stroma separating the epithelial masses.

percent differentiated cells and 75 percent immature cells. Grade 4 is the least differentiated, most anaplastic and therefore the most malignant of the four grades. Grade 4 consists of 75 percent or greater of undifferentiated cells. Grades 3 and 4, the most anaplastic neoplasms, show the best response to irradiation. The prognosis of squamous cell carcinoma is dependent upon location and grading. Squamous cell carcinoma generally has the lowest degree of malignancy when the neoplasm occurs in the lip and skin and the greatest degree of malignancy when it is located in the floor of the mouth and lateral posterior borders of the tongue.

Carcinoma in situ appears morphologically and cytologically as a carcinoma. It contains large atypical cells with hyperchromatic nuclei, numerous abnormal mitotic figures and dyskeratotic epithelium. However, the neo-

---

Figure 32 A and B. Papilloma. Notice the central connective tissue stalk with branches covered by stratified squamous epithelium. Long processes are attached to the central stalk which supports the blood vessels. The surface shows marked keratinization of the superficial epithelial cells.

←

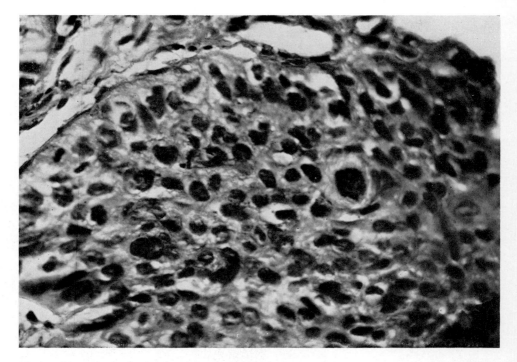

Figure 34. Carcinoma *in situ*. Notice the dyskeratosis confined to the squamous epithelium. The squamous cells demonstrate great irregularity in size and shape, hyperchromatism and abnormal mitotic figures. The basement membrane appears intact. (From Gardner, A. F.: An investigation of the use of exfoliative cytology in the diagnosis of malignant lesions of the oral cavity. The cytologic diagnosis of oral carcinoma. *Acta Cytol*, 8:436, 1964.)

plasm is confined to the epithelium of the mucous membrane and skin and has no invasive characteristics.

Basal cell carcinoma is a common malignant neoplasm of skin appendages. The basal cell carcinoma occurs on the lips and skin particularly in the nasal and cheek folds. The cure rate for the basal cell carcinoma is 100 percent because the basal cell carcinoma fails to metastasize. The initial manifestation of the basal cell carcinoma is a small waxy-appearing nodule. The center of the nodule becomes necrotic and the carcinoma subsequently consists of an ulcer bordered by a rolled indurated margin. Excessive radiation resulting from prolonged exposure to sunlight and roentgen rays are the most common etiologic factors for the development of the basal cell carcinoma.

The basal cell carcinoma is characterized histologically by masses of cells which have large deeply basophilic nuclei and minimal cytoplasm. The basal cells generally form solid masses, cysts or gland-like structures. When epithelial chords composed of basal cells undergo shrinkage with cystic degeneration the neoplasm is termed *cystic basal cell carcinoma*. The basal cell carcinoma may rarely occur mixed with the epidermoid carcinoma. The latter is termed *basosquamous cell carcinoma* of the mucous membrane.

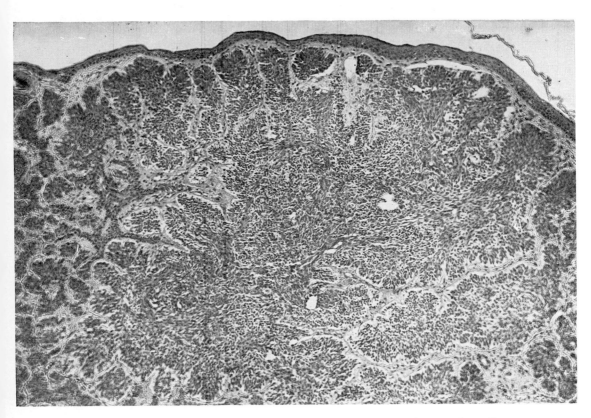

Figure 35. Basal cell carcinoma of the skin. Notice the numerous large and small masses and cords composed of deeply basophilic-stained nuclei. The cells are uniform in size, shape, and staining characteristics. The cells take a deep hematoxylin stain. Mitosis is not present. A few areas contain neoplastic cells which tend to form a glandular arrangement by surrounding a lumen.

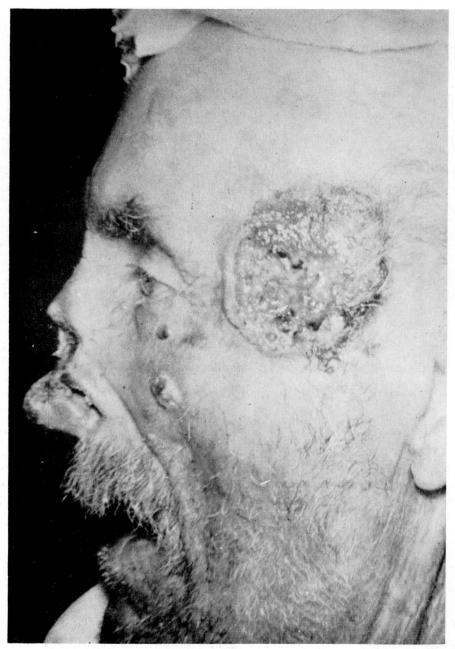

Figure 36 A and B. Basal cell carcinoma of the upper two-thirds of the face. Notice the large rodent ulcer surrounded by a raised rolled border. This carcinoma has eroded into the adjacent tissue and caused extensive local destruction of the epidermis and dermis.

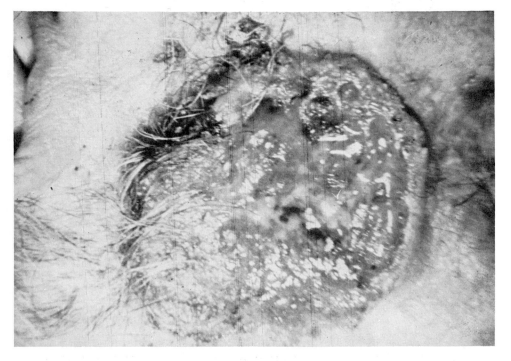

Figure 36 B.

TABLE XIII-D

Neoplasms of Mesenchymal Tissues

Cell	Benign Neoplasm	Malignant Neoplasm
Fibroblast	Fibroma	Fibrosarcoma
Chondroblast	Chondroma	Chondrosarcoma
Osteoblast	Osteoma	Osteosarcoma
Myxoblast	Myxoma	Myxosarcoma
Lipoblast	Lipoma	Liposarcoma
Notochord	Chordoma	——
Monocytic cell	Histiocytoma	——
——	Mesothelioma	Malignant Mesothelioma

Neoplasms of Epithelial Tissues

Epithelium	Benign Neoplasm	Cell	Malignant Neoplasm
Covering and lining	Papilloma	Squamous epithelial	Epidermoid carcinoma
		Transitional	Transitional cell carcinoma
		Basal	Basal cell carcinoma
Grandular-arranged in acini	Adenoma	Glandular epithelium	Adenocarcinoma

Neoplasms of Muscle Tissue

Cell	Benign Neoplasm	Malignant Neoplasm
Smooth muscle	Leiomyoma	Leiomyosarcoma
Striated muscle or skeletal muscle	Rhabdomyoma	Rhabdomyosarcoma

Neoplasms of the Vascular System

Blood vessels	Hemangioma	Hemangiosarcoma
Lymphatic vessels	Lymphangioma	Lymphangiosarcoma

Neoplasms of Endothelium

Endothelial	Endothelioma	Malignant Endothelioma

Table XIII-D (*Continued*)

Neoplasms of Peripheral Nervous Tissue

Ganglia	Ganglioneuroma (Nerve cells)	Neuroblastoma
Nerve sheath cells	Neurilemmoma	Malignant Neurilemmoma
	Neurofibroma	Neurofibrosarcoma

Neoplasms of Hematopoietic System

Cell	Benign Neoplasm	Malignant Neoplasm
Myeloid	None	Myeloid Leukemia

Neoplasms of Lymphoid Tissue

Lymphoid	Benign Lymphoma (Very Rare)	Lymphosarcoma Lymphoid Leukemia

Neoplasms of Multipotential Cells

Pluripotential cells (limited differentiation)	Mixed Tumor	Malignant Mixed Tumor
Pluripotential cells (unlimited differentiation)	Teratoma	Malignant Teratoma
Unipotential cells of three germ layers (limited differentiation)	Embryoma	——

Pigmented Neoplasms

Chromatoblast	Nevus	Malignant Melanoma

Neoplasms of the Endocrine Glands

Organ	Benign Neoplasm	Malignant Neoplasm
Thyroid	Follicular Adenoma Oxyphil Cell Adenoma	Carcinoma
Parathyroid	Adenoma	Carcinoma (rare)
Thymus	Lipoma Myxoma	Malignant Thymoma ——
Pituitary	Adenoma Craniopharyngioma	—— ——

Neoplasms of Specialized Mesoderm

Adrenal Cortex	Cortical Adenoma	Carcinoma
Kidney	——	Renal Cell Carcinoma

Neoplasms of Specialized Ectoderm

Cell	Benign Neoplasm	Malignant Neoplasm
Ameloblast	Ameloblastoma	——

Adenocarcinoma is a malignant neoplasm which arises from glandular epithelium throughout the body.

Benign Neoplasms of Mesenchymal Origin

The *fibroma* is a common benign neoplasm consisting of fibroblasts and collagenous tissue. The fibroma is a well-encapsulated neoplasm which is firm to palpation. Microscopically, the fibroblasts appear as fusiform cells between interlacing collagenous fiber bundles. A redundant mass of tissue associated with a cause and effect relationship is termed an *irritational fibroma*. *Desmoid tumor* indicates both benign and malignant fibroblastic neoplasia in muscle tissue and fascial planes. The desmoid tumor consists of well-differentiated fibroblasts and bundles of collagenous connective tis-

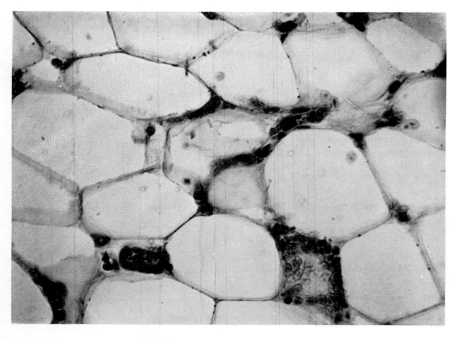

Figure 37. Lipoma. Notice the presence of fat cells very similar to the cells comprising normal adipose tissue. However, the fat cells are larger than adipose tissue cells.

sue. The desmoid tumor does not metastasize; however, it may be locally aggressive.

The *dermatofibroma protuberans* consists of several plaque-like lesions which coalesce and subsequently enlarge forming a protuberant mass of tissue in the skin. Dermatofibroma occurs in the skin and mucous membranes.

The *lipoma* is a benign neoplasm composed of mature fat tissue. The lipoma is a soft, yellow, well-circumscribed neoplasm surrounded by a connective tissue capsule. *Fibrolipomas* are composed predominantly of mature fat and a lesser quantity of fibrous connective tissue. The *myxoma* is a rare benign connective tissue neoplasm which has a local invasive characteristic. However, the myxoma does not metastasize. The myxoma consists of stellate cells and branching fusiform fibroblasts located in a loose mucoid matrix. The myxoma is a gelatinous mass which may attain a considerable size.

The *chondroma* is a rare benign neoplasm which produces cartilage following the formation of an intermediary precartilagenous tissue. The chondroma is a hard gray-colored lobulated neoplasm surrounded by a connective tissue capsule. When the chondroma occurs in bone tissue it has the capacity to attain a very large size. Sarcomatous change may occur in the chondroma: a fact that is of the utmost importance to the clinician who is going to treat the chondroma. Chondromas should be considered as potentially malignant neoplasms if they show a tendency to undergo transplantation, regardless of whether or not metastases are present. When chondromas occur in indi-

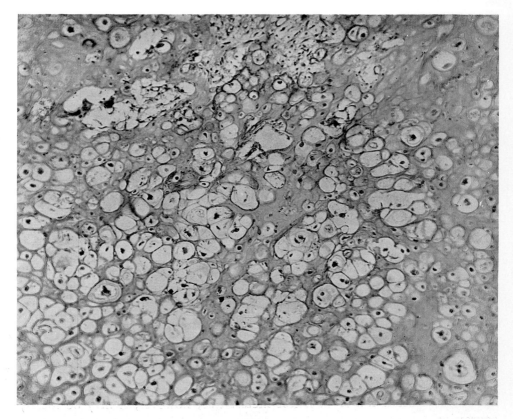

Figure 38. Chondroma. Notice the normal-appearing chondrocytes which comprise this benign mesenchymal neoplasm. The chondrocytes are separated by hyaline matrix.

viduals over nineteen years of age, they generally show a tendency toward transplantation and metastases.

True osteoma of bone tissue is a rare neoplasm. Compact osteomas of the maxilla and mandible are termed *torus palatinus* and *torus mandibularis*.

Neoplasms of Myogenic Tissue

The *leiomyoma* is a benign neoplasm of smooth muscle. Leiomyomas have the capacity to attain a large size. In rare instances, the leiomyoma may undergo malignant transformation. When removed surgically, some leiomyomas show a tendency to recur and undergo transplantation. Histopathologically, the leiomyoma consists of interlacing bundles of smooth muscle separated by minimal amounts of connective tissue. The *rhabdomyoma* is a benign muscle neoplasm derived from striated or skeletal muscle.

The *granular cell myoblastoma* is a benign neoplasm of striated muscle which occurs in the tongue, lip, larynx and esophagus. Histologically, the myoblastoma consists of large polygonal cells with highly granular cytoplasm. The origin of this neoplasm has not been established, i.e. muscular, neurogenic or fibroblastic. The *congenital epulis of the newborn* is a rare benign lesion which is morphologically similar to the granular cell myoblastoma. The congenital epulis of the newborn is located only on the gingiva of the newborn and should be classified as a distinct entity.

Benign Angiomatous Neoplasms

Hemangioma represents a new formation of blood vessels which may be difficult to distinguish from telangiectasia. *Telangiectasia* is a dilatation of pre-existing blood vessels in the skin and mucous membranes. The *capillary hemangioma* is the most common form of angioma. It is composed of a proliferation of newly-formed capillaries filled with blood. The capillary

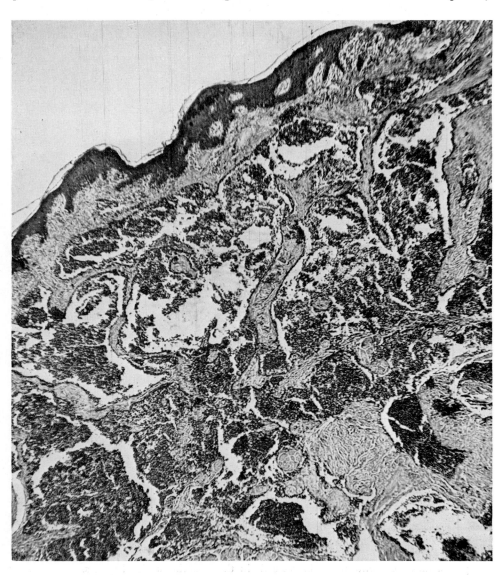

Figure 39. Cavernous hemangioma of the lip. The neoplasm is composed of numerous dilated vascular spaces or sinuses engorged with blood and lined by a single layer of endothelial cells. The surface epithelium overlying the hemangioma shows atrophic changes.

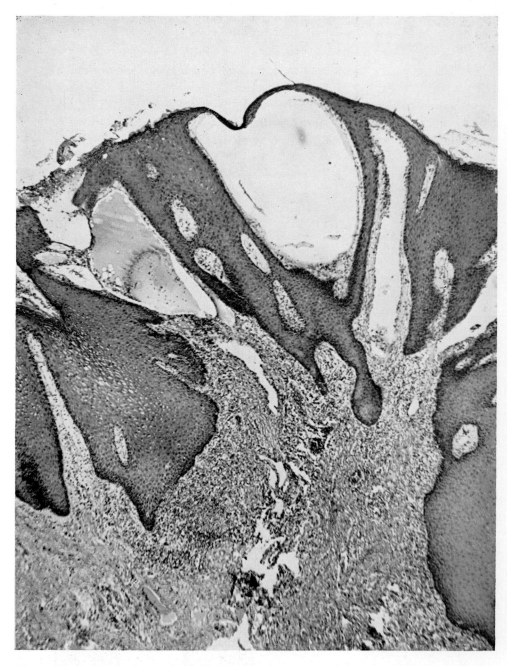

Figure 40. Lymphangioma of the lip. Notice the thin overlying stratified squamous epithelium. Beneath the epithelium are several large spaces lined by a layer of flattened endothelial cells. The lumen contains homogeneous material, i.e. lymph. The lymphangioma does not contain red blood cells in the endothelial-lined spaces.

hemangioma is a frequent cause of *macroglossia*. The hemangioma may be treated by irradiation, surgery and sclerosing solutions. *Cavernous hemangiomas* are less common than capillary hemangiomas. The cavernous hemangioma consists of large cavernous spaces lined by a single layer of thin endothelial cells. The hemangioma is not encapsulated. Cavernous hemangiomas are common in the lips.

The *lymphangioma* is a congenital angioma that occurs in both localized and diffuse forms. The lymphangioma consists of small or cavernous spaces lined by a layer of endothelium and filled with lymph. Lymphangioma is frequently the cause of *macroglossia*. The lymphangioma may be located in the lip resulting in a diffuse *macrocheilia*. When the lymphangioma occurs as a diffuse soft swelling in the neck of children, it is termed *hygroma colli cysticum*.

Malignant Neoplasms of Mesenchymal Origin

Sarcomas are malignant neoplasms arising from fibroblasts (fibrosarcoma), osteoblasts (osteosarcoma), and chondroblasts (chondrosarcoma). Sarcomas are not common neoplasms. Sarcomas generally occur before forty-five years of age. Osteogenic sarcoma occurs in individuals from twelve to thirty-five years of age. The sarcoma is a soft, fleshy mass which infiltrates the surrounding tissues. Hemorrhage is a common complication. The sar-

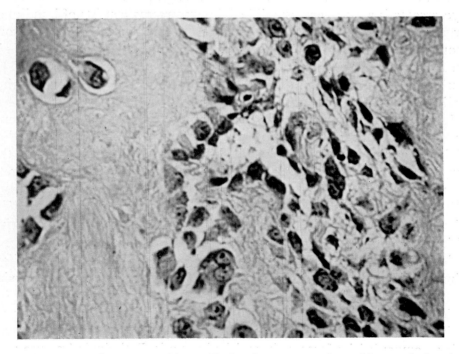

Figure 41. Osteogenic sarcoma of bone. Notice the presence of osteoblasts and abundant areas of osteoid tissue. The neoplastic osteoblasts vary in size and shape and in staining characteristics. Some neoplastic osteoblasts are small hyperchromatic cells, whereas other osteoblasts stain faintly and are rather large in size.

coma grows by expansion and infiltration. Spread of the sarcoma takes place by way of the blood stream. Tumor cell emboli develop early and metastases are produced in the lungs and visceral organs. The *fibrosarcoma* is a well-defined, soft tissue neoplasm consisting of interlacing fascicles of spindle-shaped fibroblasts and frequent mitoses.

The *osteogenic sarcoma* is composed of the osteoblast type cell; however, the most predominant portion of the neoplasm is the intercellular tissue. The osteogenic sarcoma produces two types, the *osteolytic* and *sclerotic osteogenic sarcoma*. The sclerotic osteosarcoma containing abundant bone tissue has a relatively good prognosis. The osteolytic osteogenic sarcoma containing little or no bone tissue has a relatively poor prognosis. Osteosarcomas of the jaws have a better prognosis than their counterpart in the long bones. *Chondrosarcoma* is a rare neoplasm which has a rapid growth rate. The chondrosarcoma contains numerous mitotic figures and shows great irregularity in the size and shape of neoplastic cells. The chondrosarcoma involves the sternum and pelvis more commonly than other bones.

Liposarcoma is a rare neoplasm which tends to recur after surgical excision and grows by infiltration. Microscopically, large vacuolated lipoblasts with a signet-ring morphology are arranged around a vascular network. Recurrence is common following surgery. *Myxosarcoma* is a rare sarcoma undergoing myxomatous change in focal areas. The sarcomatous connective tissue undergoes degenerative changes resulting in the myxosarcoma. *Leiomyosarcoma* is a rare neoplasm. The leiomyosarcoma consists of bundles of large elongated spindle-shaped cells. The leiomyosarcoma is a dangerous neoplasm when located in the deep tissues of the head and neck. The *rhabdomyosarcoma* is a rare neoplasm which occurs in voluntary muscle. The clinical behavior pattern of the rhabdomyosarcoma does not follow a highly malignant pattern. Metastases occur to the regional lymph nodes.

Lymphosarcoma is a malignant lymphoma of lymph nodes, spleen and bone marrow. The lymphosarcoma consists of an uncontrolled proliferation of lymphocytes resulting in lymphadenopathy. Histopathologically, the lymph node consists of uniform proliferating lymphocytes which obliterate the nodal architecture. The *reticulum cell sarcoma* is a malignant neoplasm of lymph nodes. This sarcoma is characterized by an uncontrolled proliferation of reticulum cells in lymph nodes. The reticulum cell sarcoma begins with an insidious onset of localized or generalized enlargement of lymph nodes. Histopathologically, the lymph node consists of masses of proliferating small and large reticulum cells which obliterate the normal nodal morphology. *Ewing's sarcoma* is a highly malignant neoplasm of young individuals which arises from the reticuloendothelial cells of the bone marrow. Ewing's sarcoma of bone tissue may be mistaken for osteomyelitis because it is accompanied by fever, pain and leukocytosis. Pathologic fracture may occur in the affected bone due to Ewing's sarcoma. Histopathologically, this sarcoma is composed of sheets and masses of undifferentiated small round cells located between areas of well-vascularized connective tissue.

Neoplasms of Peripheral Nervous Tissue

The *neurofibroma* is composed of a mass of tangled nerve bundles and a variable quantity of collagen. The neurofibroma may occur as an independent benign neoplasm of peripheral nervous tissue or may develop as a *generalized neurofibromatosis*. Histopathologically, the neurofibroma contains Schwann cells. This neoplasm occurs in the subcutaneous tissue along peripheral nerves as fusiform masses.

Amputation neuromas consist of proliferating nerve fibers which form bundles surrounded by an epineurium. The amputation neuroma may occur on a branch of the facial nerve or may result following trauma or severance of a peripheral nerve. The mass is movable, grows slowly and produces pain. *Plexiform neuroma* consists of a tangled mass of highly differentiated hypertrophic peripheral nerve bundles. The neoplasm may involve the facial nerve and result in a marked facial deformity. Histopathologically, numerous nerve bundles appear as a tangled mass of fascicles. When the plexiform neuroma is localized to the facial nerve it is termed *facial gigantism*. *Ganglioneuroma* is a neoplasm of peripheral nerve cells. It is a slow growing neoplasm which is composed of ganglion cells in various stages of maturation surrounded by a stroma of Schwann cells.

The *neurilemmoma* or *benign schwannoma* is a firm, well-encapsulated benign neoplasm of peripheral nervous tissue containing Antoni type A and B tissue. The Antoni type A tissue is a fasciculated or whorled area containing elongated cells and bands or zones of fibrous tissue. The nuclei of the elongated cells are arranged into a palisaded pattern. The palisaded cells surround whorls termed *Verocay bodies*. Antoni type B tissue is composed of minimal collagen fibers and irregularly dispersed cells. *Midline lethal granuloma* is a nondescriptive destructive lesion which involves the palate, nasal chambers and maxillary sinuses. The granuloma erodes bone destroying the facial bones and produces bony sequestrations, a foul odor and a greatly emaciated patient. It has a relentless clinical behavior pattern and obscure etiology. Histopathologically, the midline lethal granuloma appears as an inflammatory erosive type of lesion.

Neoplasms of Various Embryonic Tissues with a Low-grade Clinical Behavior Pattern

Embryomas. Embryomas are composed of highly differentiated cells normally present in the part. An example of the embryoma is *Wilm's tumor* of the kidney of children.

Teratomas. The teratoma is composed of cells foreign to a specific area of the body. The cells of the teratoma arise from all germ layers.

Pigmented Malignant Neoplasm

Malignant melanoma occurs in the skin and mucous membrane. It gives rise to widespread metastatic neoplasms. Melanomas may arise from a junctional or compound nevus of the skin. The prognosis of the malignant melanoma is serious. Recurrences result following failure to remove the margins of the neoplasm. Primary malignant melanoma of the mucous membrane is rare. Histopathologically, melanocarcinomatous cells infiltrate the submucosa of the skin.

Cysts and Neoplasms in the Head and Neck

Carotid Body Tumor. The carotid body tumor arises from the carotid bodies located at the bifurcation of the common carotid arteries. Histopathologically, this neoplasm is comprised of alveolar masses of polyhedral-shaped cells. The *branchial cleft cyst* produces a swelling in the lateral portion of

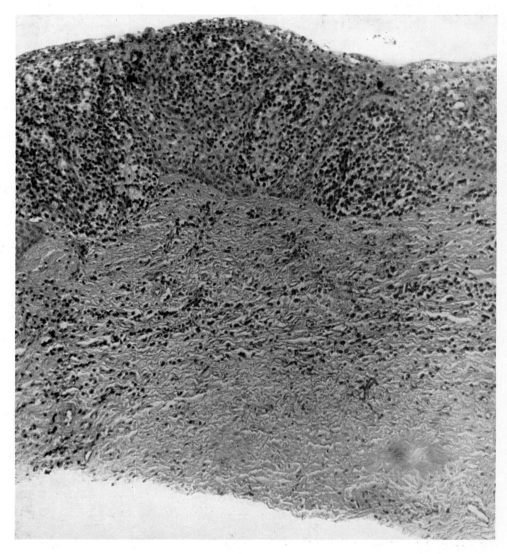

Figure 42. Microscopic appearance of the cyst wall from an epidermoid cyst of the neck. Notice the stratified squamous epithelial lining and supporting connective tissue. The epithelium and connective tissue are infiltrated by chronic inflammatory cells.

the neck anterior to the sternocleidomastoid muscle. Histopathologically, the branchial cyst is lined by stratified squamous epithelium. Lymphoid tissue and connective tissue are located beneath the epithelial lining.

The *epidermoid cyst* is lined by several layers of stratified squamous epithelium. It contains sebaceous glands, sweat glands and hair follicles in the wall of the cyst. The *dermoid cyst* is a variant of the epidermoid cyst. The connective tissue wall of the cyst may contain hair follicles, sebaceous glands, sweat glands, striated muscle and mucous glands.

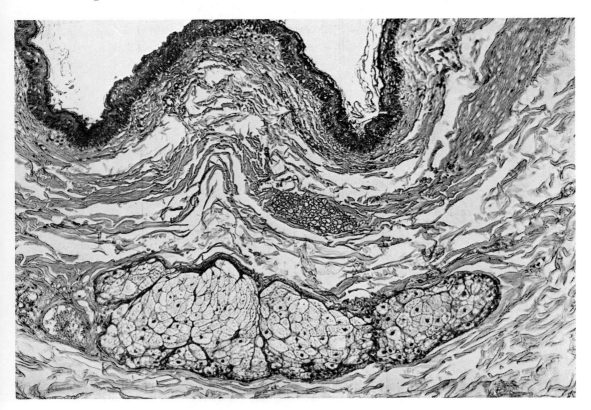

Figure 43. Dermoid cyst. Notice that the cyst wall is lined by keratinized squamous epithelium and the connective tissue wall contains sebaceous glands. Hair follicles may also be present. The lining of this dermoid cyst is rough and irregular.

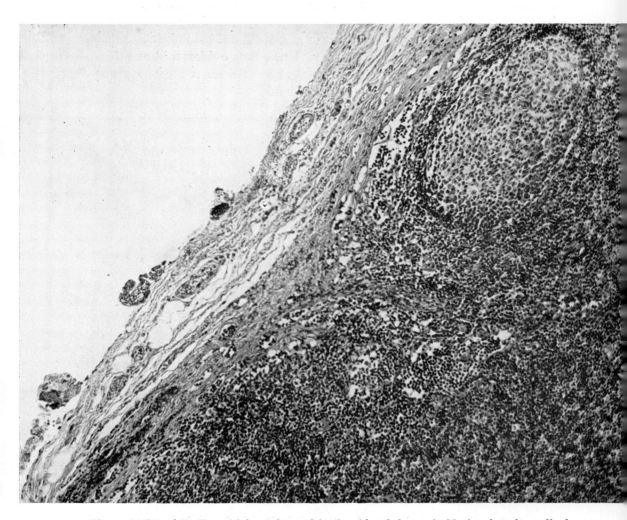

Figure 44 A and B. Branchial cyst located in the side of the neck. Notice that the wall of the cyst is denuded of stratified squamous epithelium. Beneath the epithelium and connective tissue is lymphoid tissue containing large germinal centers. The presence of lymphoid tissue in the cyst wall is characteristic of the branchial cyst.

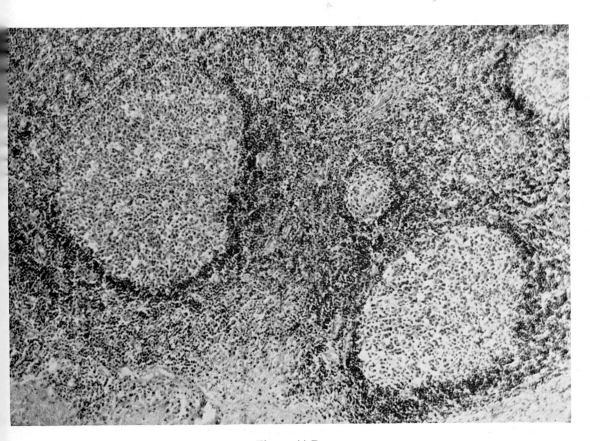

Figure 44 **B.**

Chapter 9

HYPERSENSITIVITY AND DISEASES OF CONNECTIVE TISSUE

HYPERSENSITIVITY

*H*ypersensitivity* or *allergy* is the study of specific reactions occurring between antigens and antibodies resulting in pathologic effects on tissues. An *antigen* is a substance capable of evoking an antibody response *in vivo*. An *antibody* is a substance capable of combining specifically with an antigen against which it is directed. The alterations in cells may be due to the presence of toxic substances resulting from the antigen-antibody reaction.

Immediate Hypersensitivity. *Immediate hypersensitivity* results in a reaction within seconds to minutes following the exposure to an antigen in the sensitive patient. The manifestations of the immediate type of hypersensitivity include the following basic characteristics: a rapid response, reactivity of antibody of the blood, and secondarily the participation of cells in the antigen-antibody reaction. The *Arthus phenomenon* and anaphylactic type reactions are examples of immediate hypersensitivity. In the Arthus phenomenon precipitating antibodies having good reactivity combine with the antigen in the tissues and produce injury to vascular endothelium. The first injection of an antigen produces no effect. However, the second injection of the antigen may be accompanied, within a half-hour, by edema which persists for several hours. Subsequent injections result in more pronounced edema until eventually the reaction progresses to necrosis.

Delayed Hypersensitivity. *Delayed hypersensitivity* requires more than a single exposure to the same antigen. The initial dose of antigen does not produce an observable response for twenty-four to seventy-two hours which may persist for days. The reactive tissue of delayed hypersensitivity is the portal of entry of the antigenic stimulus, i.e. the mucous membrane or skin. *Dermatitis venenata* occurs in the sensitized individual following contact with noninfectious substances. Many drugs may provoke contact forms of delayed hypersensitivity. Repeated exposure to the offending substance results in a contact dermatitis, delayed hypersensitivity.

Anaphylaxis. Anaphylaxis is an acute reaction which may occur following the injection of antigens into hypersensitive individuals. In anaphylaxis a small amount of nonprecipitating or precipitating antibodies are required to produce the shock-like reaction. Anaphylaxis is a hypersensitivity of the immediate type. If the antigen is injected intravenously, anaphylaxis may result. Very small doses of antigen will produce the anaphylactic state. *Anaphylactic shock* is a sequence of events which begins in seconds following the introduction of the antigen. The findings include smooth muscle contraction, edema, fall in blood pressure, general leukopenia and thrombocytopenia.

CONNECTIVE TISSUE DISEASES

Connective tissue diseases or the *collagen diseases* are characterized by systemic involvement of the connective tissues throughout the body. The diseases of connective tissue reflect a local response of a particular tissue to irritants or injurious agents. In addition to deposition of fibrinoid material, the connective tissue diseases show the following changes: mucoid degeneration, fibrosis and hyalinization when healing occurs in the fibrinoid material.

Systemic or Disseminated Lupus Erythematosus. Disseminated lupus erythematosus is an acute, subacute and recurrent febrile disease occurring principally in women. The disease produces widespread involvement of the connective tissue throughout the body. The following features may be present during the course of the disease: erythematous rash on the face; renal, gastrointestinal and central nervous system involvement; joint pain and swelling; proteinuria; cardiac involvement; lymphadenopathy; fever, anemia, and thrombocytopenia. The most important etiologic factor in systemic lupus erythematosus is hypersensitivity to an antigen. The blood vessels show advanced fibrinoid degeneration in systemic lupus. The thickened basement membrane of glomerular capillary tufts becomes smudgy due to eosinophilic deposits of fibrinoid material, i.e. *wire loop lesions.*

The lupus erythematosus cells (L.E. cells) appear to be polymorphonuclear neutrophilic leukocytes which have engulfed large basophilic hematoxylin bodies. The L.E. cell is not pathognomonic for disseminated lupus erythematosus. In the joints, proliferation of the synovial membrane produces arthritis. Disseminated lupus erythematosus is exacerbated by exposure to sunlight. A skin rash is present in approximately 80 percent of affected individuals. The most characteristic skin lesion is an erythematous local maculopapular rash distributed over the bridge of the nose and cheek, producing a butterfly lesion on the face.

Chronic Discoid Lupus Erythematosus. A form of lupus erythematosus is limited to the skin termed *chronic discoid lupus erythematosus.*

Scleroderma. Scleroderma is a rare chronic systemic connective tissue disease in which the skin and mucous membrane become thickened and stiff due to excessive collagenization. Two forms of scleroderma are recognized —morphea (localized lesion) and diffuse (generalized lesions). The dermatologic and mucous membrane changes constitute the most visible alterations. An indurated skin develops which is adherent to the atrophic subcutaneous tissue. Induration is followed by atrophic changes in the

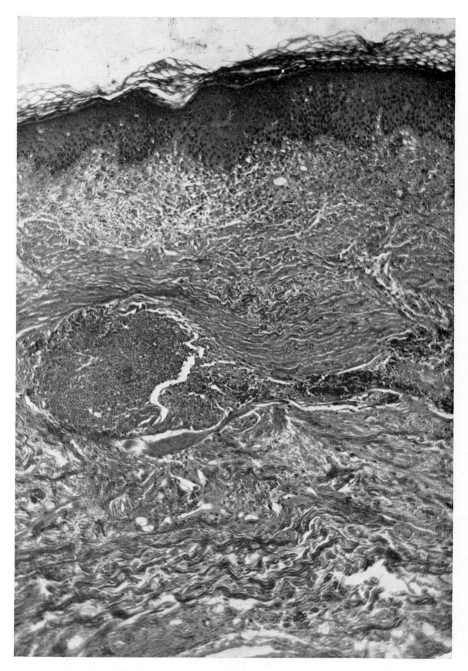

Figure 45. Chronic discoid lupus erythematosus of the skin. Notice the hyperkeratosis, increased thickness of the granular cell layer, alternating areas of acanthosis and epithelial atrophy, and the flattened rete ridges. A patchy inflammatory infiltrate is present. The hair follicles have degenerated and are therefore not visible in this section. The elastica and collagen bundles have undergone degenerative changes.

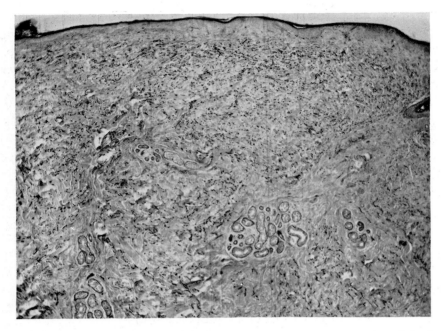

Figure 46. Scleroderma of the skin. Notice the fibrous proliferation (fibrosis) of the dermis and narrowing and obliteration of small arterioles. Atrophic changes are present in the overlying epithelium and skin appendages.

epithelium, and connective tissue producing a shiny, smooth and fixed skin containing irregular areas of pigmentation. The main alteration in scleroderma is hyalinization of the connective tissue.

Polyarteritis Nodosa. Polyarteritis is a subacute or chronic necrotizing inflammation involving all layers of the walls of medium and small arteries, arterioles and capillaries. The disease is characterized by a low-grade fever, arthralgia, muscular tenderness, skin eruptions and central nervous system, renal and cardiac alterations. The first stage consists of edema, and fibrinoid and mucoid degeneration beginning in the media and extending to the adventitia and intima of medium and small arteries and arterioles. The second stage is characterized by an inflammatory infiltrate of polymorphonuclear leukocytes involving all layers of the vessel wall and perivascular tissues. The third stage is characterized by proliferation of fibroblasts and endothelial cells and formation of granulation tissue. The fourth stage consists of resolution of the inflammatory infiltrate with formation of dense fibrous connective tissue.

Dermatomyositis. Dermatomyositis is a rare connective tissue disease involving the skin and skeletal muscles which is characterized by a sudden onset and acute rapid course. The findings include edema and erythematous rashes involving the face, neck, periorbital region, extremities and trunk; arthralgia; myalgia; muscle weakness; fever and peripheral neuritis.

Serum Sickness. Serum sickness is a form of hypersensitivity which generally subsides spontaneously. The manifestations of serum sickness may appear without any prior sensitization to an antigen. The manifestations are fever, urticaria, adenopathy, edema and joint pain. Arthritis commonly accompanies patients with serum sickness. Generalized lymphadenopathy and edema of the eyelids, glottis, hands, and feet are manifestations of serum sickness.

Chapter 10

RADIATION INJURY TO TISSUES AND DEFICIENCY DISEASES

RADIATION INJURY TO TISSUES

Cellular Changes during Radiation. *Radiosensitive tissues* include those tissues in which 2500 roentgens or less will produce death or injury. The latter group includes lymphocytes, gastrointestinal tract epithelium, bone marrow and germ cells. *Radioresponsive tissues* include those tissues which are killed or injured by 2500 to 5000 roentgens. The latter group includes mucous membrane, skin and epidermal appendages, salivary glands, endothelium, growing bone and cartilage, conjunctiva, cornea and lens, collagen and elastic tissue. *Radioresistant tissues* include those tissues which are killed or injured by over 5000 roentgens. The latter group includes kidneys, liver, thyroid, pancreas, pituitary, adrenal, muscle, nerves and mature bone.

Cellular Differentiation. The more highly specialized cells are less affected by radiation than the undifferentiated cells. Radiation has an accumulative effect but not total summation. When a tissue is irradiated for the initial time, healing occurs promptly. During reirradiation of the tissue, one-half the dose produces the same effect as a full dose of the initial radiation.

Systemic Effects of Radiation. *Radiation sickness* (first phase) occurs in a few hours to three days following irradiation. Nausea, vomiting, depression, shock, and an acute self-limited illness develops. The second phase is *radiation cachexia*. The individual develops an apathetic state with loss of weight, depression, general wasting and death. The second phase appears in three weeks or in three months. The altered metabolism causes a depression of antibodies, therefore secondary infection may occur in the irradiated tissues.

General Effects of Irradiation on Tissues. Vacuolation of the nucleus is followed by vacuolated cytoplasm, swelling of cells, edema, sloughing of epithelium, dilatation, hemangiectasia, conversion of the connective tissue into an amorphous structure, and permeability and rupture of vessel walls are generalized effects.

Irradiated tissue has an impaired ability for regeneration and repair. Bacterial invasion becomes prevalent following irradition damage to mucous membrane and skin. The effects of radiation occur primarily in the veins and lymphatics. Irradiated bones are brittle and pathologic fractures may result. Local necrosis and *aseptic necrosis of bone* are the causes of pathologic fractures following irradiation of bone tissue. Bone tissue of the jaw is exposed to small quantities of irradiation in individuals employed in industries where radioactive radium dials are manufactured. The latter irradiation may result in the formation of osteogenic sarcoma of the jaw.

Radioactive Contamination. The daily allowable radiation is 0.1 roentgen per day or 0.3 roentgen per week. Eight hundred roentgens given as a total body exposure will kill an individual. Radiation dermatitis occurs following exposure to 600 to 800 roentgens. Leukemia is three to four times greater in radiologists than in the remainder of the medical profession.

Radioactive Isotopes in Research. All radioactive isotopes decay; however, beta rays, positrons, and gamma rays ionize the matter through which they pass. The major areas of radioactive isotope research involve testing the uptake and permeability of various cells and tissues with special reference to physiologic exchange of substances.

TISSUE RESPONSES TO DEFICIENCY DISEASES

Nutritional Disease Syndromes in Man

Hypokaliemia produces morphologic alterations in tissues. Insufficient intake of animal protein results in *kwashiorkor*. The manifestations of this nutritional deficiency are anemia, low plasma protein level, loose bowels, edema around the eyes and on the hand, arms, legs and feet, and depigmentation of the skin. Excessive insulin produces a deficiency of carbohydrates. Deficiency of fat is due to poor absorption during biliary disease.

Vitamin A Deficiency

The initial manifestation of vitamin A deficiency is *night blindness*. A lesion resulting from avitaminosis A is squamous metaplasia of columnar and transitional epithelium to keratinizing squamous epithelium. Hyperkeratosis of the skin and mucous membranes is due to vitamin A deficiency. Vitamin A deficiency causes atrophy of cartilage and bone and reduces the normal resistance of the tissues to infections.

Hypervitaminosis A. Hypervitaminosis A accelerates degeneration and maturation of cartilage and the remodeling of bone tissue resulting in multiple fractures.

Vitamin B Complex Deficiency

Vitamin B_1 or thiamine deficiency produces the *beriberi syndrome.* Three clinical types of beriberi have been recognized—*dry beriberi* producing neurological involvement, *cardiac beriberi* producing heart failure, and *wet beriberi* producing generalized edema and anasarca. Beriberi is associated with a diet composed mainly of polished rice. A burning feet syndrome is prevalent in prisoners of war who have beriberi. They experience burning feet, with extreme pain in the feet and lower extremities.

Riboflavin or vitamin B₂ deficiency produces prominent alterations in the mucous membranes and skin. The tongue becomes enlarged, red to purple in color, with a smooth surface, i.e. *magenta glossitis*. Dermatitis with hyperkeratosis, cheilosis with fissuring at the corners of the mouth, conjunctivitis and visual disturbances are symptoms of riboflavin deficiency. *Nicotinic acid deficiency* produces *pellagra*. A scrotal dermatitis develops during pellagra. A single nutritional deficiency resulting from riboflavin, nicotinic acid, or pyridoxine deficiency all produce a similar *scrotal dermatitis. Pyridoxine (vitamin B₆) deficiency* produces abdominal pain, weakness on exertion, but is reversed by administering pyridoxine. A pure *pantothenic acid deficiency* does not exist in man. *Biotin deficiency* may rarely produce dermatitis, muscle pains, nausea and anemia.

In *pernicious anemia* the mucosa of the stomach is atrophic and contains

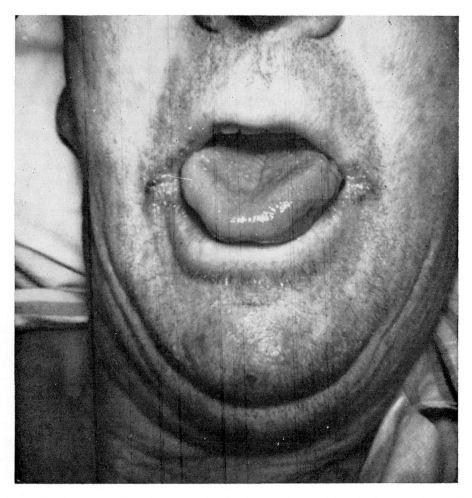

Figure 47. Glossitis and cheilosis associated with riboflavin (vitamin B₂) deficiency. Notice the cracks and fissures at the angles of the mouth (cheilosis) and the inflammation of the tongue (glossitis).

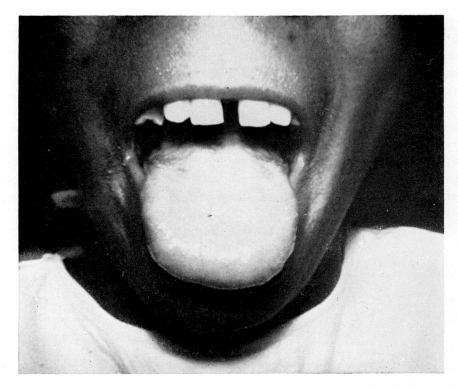

Figure 48. Pellagra affecting the tongue. Notice the red, swollen and sore tongue associated with pellagra. Ulceration of the tongue eventually takes place following a long-standing deficiency of nicotinic acid. Histopathologic findings reveal similar changes in the skin and oral mucosa.

a cellular infiltrate of lymphocytic cells. During pernicious anemia there is an absence of free hydrochloric acid in the gastric juice because the atrophic gastric mucosa fails to secrete hydrochloric acid or pepsin. Vitamin B_{12} fails to be absorbed by the atrophic gastric mucosa. The *intrinsic factor* is a material secreted by the fundus of the stomach to facilitate the absorption of vitamin B_{12} through the upper gastrointestinal tract. Deficiency of vitamin B_{12} may occur due to increased excretion or increased demand during megaloblastic anemia of pregnancy or infancy. Pernicious anemia produces alterations in erythropoietic tissue and nervous tissue.

Vitamin C Deficiency

Vitamin C deficiency produces a single nutritional disease in infants and adults. Petechiae and perifollicular hemorrhages occur around hair follicles. Vitamin C is intimately associated with the integrity of the endothelial cementing substance, and it affects the metabolism of fibroblasts, odontoblasts and osteoblasts. Vitamin C is necessary to maintain the integrity of the intercellular substance of connective tissue, osteoid, and bone. Vitamin

C deficiency is responsible for the failure in the laying down of a normal matrix.

Scurvy results when vitamin C deficiency is severe and prolonged. The affected individuals have diffuse subcutaneous hemorrhages, anemia and edema. In children with scurvy there is decreased bone growth and alterations in the formation of the dentition. The manifestations of scurvy are pronounced in the growing bones and developing teeth. Bone trabeculae in the long bones, maxilla, and mandible are thin and inhibited in their normal growth pattern. The cortex of bones is thin due to the lack of collagen and osteoid matrix. Fractures may occur in the abnormal bone trabeculae of long bones.

Vitamin D Deficiency

Vitamin D deficiency in humans leads to the development of rickets in children and osteomalacia in adults. *Rickets* is a disease of infants and young children (under two years of age) characterized by a failure in the deposition of calcium and phosphate in the osteoid matrix. An abundant formation of osteoid tissue occurs during rickets. Although increased osteoblastic activity is evident during rickets, calcification is absent. Rickets is accompanied by the following features: rachitic rosary; bossing of the frontal and parietal bones; funneled chest; bowlegs; knock-knees; widened epiphyseal plate; osteoid tissue formation in metaphysis; and softening and bending of long bones. Infants and children with rickets have a decreased serum calcium, decreased serum phosphorus and increased serum alkaline phosphatase. Fractures may occur because of the deformities of bone tissue. When vitamin D is given in therapeutic doses, the osteoid tissue undergoes mineralization and remodelling takes place.

Osteomalacia occurs in adults during vitamin D deficiency. In osteomalacia the mature bones undergo demineralization with bowing of the lower extremities. The serum calcium and phosphorus are decreased and the serum alkaline phosphatase is increased. *Vitamin D resistant rickets* is a disease primarily of mineralized tissues. The administration of vitamin D has no therapeutic effect. The serum calcium and phosphorus levels are normal and the serum alkaline phosphatase is elevated.

Hypervitaminosis D. Excessive intake of vitamin D results in osteosclerosis and anemia. The marrow spaces are replaced by bone trabeculae.

Vitamin K Deficiency

Occasionally patients on prolonged antibiotic therapy will have a deficiency of vitamin K because the antibiotic destroys the intestinal flora which is producing vitamin K.

Vitamin E Deficiency

There have been no reports of avitaminosis E or hypervitaminosis E in man.

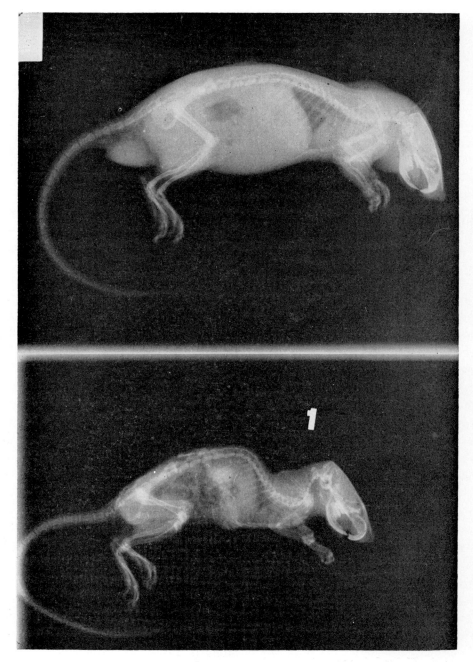

Figure 49. Hypervitaminosis D. Notice that the top radiograph represents a control litter-mate rat. The bottom radiograph shows a representative animal taken from a group of rats following subcutaneous injections of high doses of vitamin D_3 hydrosol. Notice that the anterior curvature of the dorsal spine is markedly increased. (From Gardner, A. F.: Severe spinal curvature in rats injected with a water-dispersible vitamin D_3 preparation. *Toxic Appl Pharmacol,* 8:438, 1966.)

Chapter 11

DISEASES OF THE HEART AND BLOOD VESSELS

DEGENERATIVE DISEASES OF THE HEART

Postmortem **Changes.** Postmortem changes in the heart are termed *rigor mortis*. Stiffness begins in the heart one hour after death. The left ventricle is the first chamber of the heart involved with rigor mortis. In twenty-four hours the heart is flat and the stiffness disappears.

Disturbances of Protein Metabolism. Cloudy swelling, hydropic degeneration, hyaline droplet degeneration, and primary amyloidosis are the degenerative disturbances of protein metabolism which affect the heart. The heart is involved along with the mesenchymal tissues of the body during primary amyloidosis. Amyloid may be deposited in muscle fibers of the media of the coronary arteries.

Disturbances of Fat Metabolism. *Fatty infiltration or fatty ingrowth of the myocardium* may occur in the heart particularly in the right ventricle during starvation and debilitating diseases. Fat grows into the myocardium, separates the cardiac muscle fibers, and produces atrophy of cardiac muscle fibers. Fatty ingrowth is very common in the right ventricle. A normal heart can control output; however, a heart with fatty infiltration or ingrowth is embarrassed. Pneumonia plus an embarrassed right ventricle due to fatty ingrowth may lead to an absence of resolution and death. *Fatty change or fatty degeneration* occurs within cardiac muscle fibers due to anemia and anoxia of cardiac muscle fibers. Streaks occur in the myocardium as a result of fatty change or degeneration. The latter streaks are termed *tiger striped heart.*

Disturbances in Carbohydrate Metabolism. *Von Gierke's glycogen storage disease* produces an enlarged heart due to glycogen accumulation. The latter destroys cardiac muscle fibers. Von Gierke's disease may be localized or generalized.

Disturbances of Calcification. Dystrophic calcification occurs in areas of cardiac fiber necrosis. Metastatic calcification is present in the normal myocardium during hyperparathyroidism and hypervitaminosis D.

Nutritional Deficiencies. Starvation results in atrophy of the heart. The heart is small and brown in color during starvation. The latter is termed *brown atrophy* of the heart. The brown color is due to glycofuchsin pigment which is the result of a degenerative process in cardiac muscle fibers. Vitamin B_1 (thiamine) deficiency causes alterations in cardiac muscle due to the production of beriberi. During beriberi the heart is enlarged, the right side of the heart is dilated, and there is an accumulation of fluid within and between cardiac muscle fibers. Subpericardial hemorrhage, hemopericardium, and cardiac tamponade (compression of the heart) all may result from a rare vitamin C deficiency in the United States.

ENDOCARDITIS

Rheumatic Fever (Rheumatic Endocarditis). Rheumatic fever is a systemic collagen disease which involves all layers of the heart, i.e. a pancarditis. Rheumatic fever generally occurs in children ranging from five to fifteen years of age. It has a somewhat higher incidence in females than males. The disease is more common in the temperate zone, rainy climates, and where sudden changes in temperature take place. It has a higher incidence in the lower socioeconomic populations. The greater susceptibility in the poor population is related to poor nutrition and poor resistance.

Rheumatic fever results from a poststreptococcal sensitization from group A hemolytic streptococci. The disease follows a streptococcal infection in the upper respiratory tract. There is involvement of the valves and the endocardium. The mitral and aortic valves are affected in 40 percent and only the aortic valve in 10 percent of the instances of rheumatic fever. Collagen degeneration produces a focus of degenerating tissue causing a bulging of the involved area of the mitral and aortic valves. Therefore, small wart-like elevations termed *verrucae* develop at the line of closure of the affected mitral and aortic valves and only rarely of the affected tricuspid and pulmonary valves. The verrucae are attached and cannot be wiped off of the valve leaflets at autopsy. When healing occurs stenosis and insufficiency are present in the involved valves. The entire mitral and aortic valves and endocardium are involved in the advanced stage of rheumatic fever. The affected portions of the endocardium have gross white elevations termed *McCallum's plaque*. The myocardium is grossly dilated with hypertrophy of the heart chambers directly related to the specific affected valves. If the mitral valve is involved, the left auricle becomes grossly dilated following endocardial involvement. Therefore, the heart chamber behind the involved valve undergoes dilatation during rheumatic fever. Both stenosis and insufficiency take place during rheumatic fever. The pericardium shows an acute fibrinous inflammation and contains an exudate of fibrin, inflammatory cells and fluid. The pericardial surfaces may be completely fused when healing occurs following organization of the acute fibrinous pericarditis.

The diagnostic lesions of rheumatic fever are areas of collagen necrosis termed *Aschoff bodies* located in the vicinity of the myocardial blood vessels. The collagen necrosis (fibrinoid necrosis) is accompanied by histiocytes and mononuclear cells located perivascularly in connective tissue between cardiac muscle fibers. True aschoff bodies are principally located in the atrial myocardium. One must find aschoff bodies with fibrinoid degeneration before rheumatic heart disease is definitely established histopathologically.

Complications of rheumatic fever include the following: arteries adjacent to the adrenals and arterial supply of the brain show proliferative verrucous arteritis (wart-like lesions project into the arteries); collagen necrosis in joints; proliferation of the endothelium of glomerular tufts in the kidneys without resulting in renal failure; pleuritis; interstitial pneumonitis; organized bronchopneumonia; mural thrombi on the wall of the left auricle; and embolism and infarction in the spleen and kidney.

TABLE XIV

DIFFERENTIATING FEATURES OF RHEUMATIC FEVER

MacCallum plaque on wall of left auricle
Fishmouth mitral valve with calcified leaflets
Aschoff bodies
Anitschkow cells
Bread and butter pericarditis
Thickened and curled aortic leaflets
Mild patchy pericarditis
Fibrinoid degeneration of C.T. in subendocardium
Verrucous vegetations on aortic and mitral valves
Shortening of chordae tendinae
Mitral and aortic valves affected

Endocarditis Associated With Disseminated Lupus Erythematosus. Lupus erythematosus associated with endocarditis is termed *Liebman Sachs endocarditis,* i.e. a veruccous endocarditis. Grossly, the veruccae are located anywhere on the valve leaflets and on the mural endocardium. Collagen necrosis occurs in the myocardium but Aschoff bodies are absent in endocarditis with lupus erythematosus. Vascular involvement occurs in the small and medium sized arterioles and in the heart during lupus erythematosus. Lupus is therefore characterized by the following features: (1) wire loop kidney, (2) hematoxylin bodies in the blood vessels of the ovaries and serous surfaces, and (3) endocardial involvement or Liebman Sachs endocarditis. A substance is present in the serum of individuals with lupus which causes segmented leukocytes termed the *LE cell.*

BACTERIAL ENDOCARDITIS

Subacute Bacterial Endocarditis. Subacute bacterial endocarditis is due to bacteria of low virulence, i.e. *Streptococcus viridans* or *Hemophilus influenza.* Patients may survive for extended periods of time. Previously damaged heart valves are infected by microorganisms of low virulence. The result is the formation of large gray nodular vegetations which are neither soft nor extremely firm to palpation. The vegetations are firmly attached to the valve leaflets which have been previously injured by a prior disease. The large vegetations consist of fibrin, leukocytes and bacterial colonies.

Acute Bacterial Endocarditis. Acute bacterial endocarditis occurs in the third, fourth and fifth decades of life. Vegetations develop on valves which were *not* previously damaged or altered by disease. The vegetations are rather large and poorly attached to the valve; therefore, they are readily dislodged. Dislodgement leads to septic emboli which terminate in distant organs and are responsible for the spread of the endocarditis. No organization takes place in the vegetation; therefore, it is not adherent to the valve. The most common microorganisms causing acute bacterial endocarditis are *Staphylococcus albus,* pneumococcus, streptococci, *Pseudomonas aeruginosa* and *Aerobactus aerogenes.* Acute bacterial endocarditis may accompany any acute bacterial or fungal disease. Patients with acute bacterial endocarditis develop a septic myocarditis with abscesses within the myocardium.

The septic emboli which develop in acute bacterial endocarditis lodge in the spleen, kidney and brain. Acute bacterial endocarditis leads to the formation of mycotic aneurysms in various vessels, petechial hemorrhage in the fingers, and local embolic phenomenon. Acute bacterial endocarditis produces alterations in the left ventricle and mitral valve. A mass is present on the wall of the atrium containing bacteria. The latter is an infected thrombus; however, because it occurs in the region of the heart valve it is termed a *vegetation*.

In acute bacterial endocarditis the patient may develop a pneumonia and succumb because of an absence of lung tissue or death may be due to a bacteremia or septicemia. A pyemia with minute abscesses may occur in various organs of the body because of the action of the heart valve.

In anomalies of the heart in which a patent ductus arteriosus is present, bacteria will often localize in the region of the ductus arteriosus causing an inflammation indentical with a heart valve inflammation. The patent ductus arteriosus predisposes the heart to acute bacterial endocarditis. Malformations of heart valves may also become the site of acute bacterial endocarditis.

Syphilitic Aortic Valvulitis. Syphilis produces changes in the aortic valve and damages the *vasa vasorum* of the aorta. A proliferative aortitis results with obliteration of the lumen and perivascular cuffing (the presence of plasma cells and other inflammatory cells surrounding the periphery of vessels) . The *vasa vasorum* proliferate and infiltrate into the media destroying it. An aneurysm develops following destruction of the media.

Myocarditis. Myocarditis results from rheumatic fever, acute bacterial endocarditis, acute infectious diseases, measles, diphtheria, scarlet fever, typhoid fever, Rocky Mountain spotted fever, typhus, pneumonia, gonorrhea and poliomyelitis. Diphtheria produces a diffuse interstitial myocarditis. Scarlet fever produces myocarditis due to involvement of small arterioles. Typhoid fever causes focal or acute myocarditis. Rocky Mountain spotted fever and typhus produce a myocarditis following involvement of the endothelial lining of blood vessels. Pneumonia may produce a pneumococcal myocarditis or endocarditis. Gonorrhea causes a gonococcal myocarditis. Pneumonia and gonorrhea affect the valves of the right side of the heart. Pyogenic cocci, rickettsia and other bacteria may cause a myocarditis. During uremia, the myocardium is markedly edematous and infiltrated with focal interstitial mononuclear cells. The latter changes are termed *uremic myocarditis.* Parasites and leishmaniasis evoke myocarditis. Various helminths (worms) enter the heart resulting in a myocarditis.

Pericarditis. Involvement of the pericardium as well as all layers of the heart occurs in uremia. Uremic pericarditis is a fibrinous pericarditis involving the visceral and parietal layers. A diffuse or localized pericarditis results from damaged cardiac muscle. Pericarditis occurs over an infarction of the heart.

Bacterial pericarditis may be secondary to trauma with invasion of the blood stream by microorganisms. Pneumococcal pericarditis occurs following lobar pneumonia. Tubercular pericarditis is due to an extension of the infection from the lung or the result of miliary tuberculosis. In chronic pericarditis a long-standing inflammation followed by repair results in adhesions between the parietal and visceral pericardium producing constrictive pericarditis. In chronic cases of pericarditis, fibrosis and calcification may take place. The latter change is termed *calcific pericarditis* and is visible as a radiopacity on the roentgenogram.

CONGENITAL ANOMALIES OF THE HEART

Anomalies may be diagnosed by catheterization of the heart. A catheter is placed through a vein and enters the heart. The oxygen content of the blood is determined in the atrium, ventricle, and pulmonary artery to determine whether arterial or venous blood is present and therefore whether an anomaly exists.

Patent Foramen Ovale. A patent foramen ovale is responsible for a mixture of venous and arterial blood since venous blood passes from the right to the left auricle.

Abnormalities in Septation. When the ventricular septum fails to form, the heart consists of two auricles and one ventricle. The latter is termed *cor triloculare.* When the atrial septum fails to form the heart consists of one auricle and two ventricles. The latter is termed *cor biventriculare.*

Transposition Complexes. The *tetralogy of Fallot* represents a combination of four anomalies of the heart, i.e. a patent interventricular septum, pulmonary stenosis, hypertrophy of the right ventricle, and displacement of the aorta to the right so that it arises over the patent interventricular septum. *Eisenmenger's complex* represents a combination of three defects, i.e. hypertrophy of the right ventricle, interventricular septal defect, and transposition of the aorta.

Patent Ductus Arteriosus. If the ductus arteriosus remains open after birth, blood is shunted to the pulmonary artery from the aorta. The patent ductus arteriosus can be corrected surgically.

Coarctation of the Aorta. Coarctation of the aorta is a narrowing of the aorta below the insertion of the ductus arteriosus in adults and between the origin of the left subclavian artery and ductus arteriosus in infants. Decreased blood flow stimulates the development of a compensatory collateral circulation.

DISEASES OF ARTERIES

The two most important diseases today are pathologic blood vessels and neoplasia. Approximately one-third of the individuals over forty-five years of age have some form of disease of the blood vessels. Seventy percent of the population over seventy years of age have senile coronary insufficiency. Seventy percent of individuals with diabetes who survive twenty years show evidence of atherosclerosis. Approximately 30 percent of the population over forty-five years of age die of atherosclerosis.

Degenerative Diseases of Arteries. *Arteriosclerosis* is a term referring to thickening and hardening of the arteries. The following alterations to blood vessels are included in the use of the latter term, i.e. atherosclerosis, medial sclerosis, and arteriolar sclerosis. *Atherosclerosis* is a thickening and degeneration of the intima and primarily of the large elastic vessels, i.e. the aorta. Atherosclerosis is the only form of arteriosclerosis which predisposes the artery to thrombosis. When large quantities of lipids are deposited in the intima, the intima becomes thickened. Any pathologic process in or near the intima will secondarily cause an increase in connective tissue with fibrosis and sclerosis leading to atherosclerosis. Atherosclerosis shows large lipoid deposits between the intima and media.

Atherosclerosis is related to cholesterol and the lipids present in the blood stream. The dietary intake of cholesterol by individuals consuming high quantities of eggs, animal fat, and dairy products appears to be related to the incidence of atherosclerosis.

Mönckeberg's medial calcification or sclerosis is a form of arteriosclerosis affecting the muscular arteries of the extremities. The medium-sized arteries of the extremities are elongated and a degenerative change occurs confined to the media with deposition of calcium salts in a ring-like fashion in the media. Upon palpation the artery affected by Mönckeberg's sclerosis feels like a rigid tube. Calcium salts are deposited in the necrotic tissue of the media and the artery becomes hard and brittle; however, the lumen is not narrowed and thrombosis does not occur.

Arteriolar sclerosis occurs in small arteries and precapillary vessels, and is characterized by the following changes: intimal hyalinization, hypertrophy of the media, degeneration of the media, and proliferation of the intima. Arteriolar sclerosis occurs most frequently in the afferent arterioles of the kidneys, central arterioles of the spleen and the arterioles of the pancreas, adrenal, and retina. Benign hypertension produces arteriolar sclerosis in the kidney and retina.

Coronary Arteriosclerosis and Myocardial Infarction. Coronary arteriosclerosis occurs in a degenerative form of the disease when cholesterol is deposited in the intima. The thickened intima may also be replaced by hy-

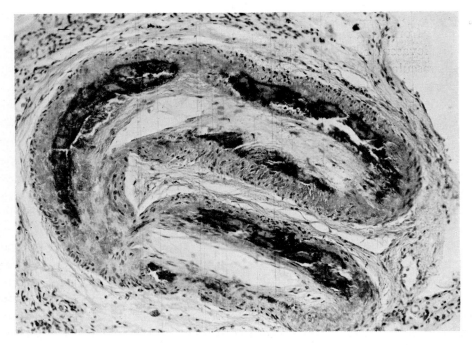

Figure 50. Medial sclerosis of an artery (Mönckeberg's sclerosis). Notice the calcified material located in the media of the artery. The calcification is preceded by degeneration of the muscle fibers of the media.

alinized connective tissue and calcification, i.e. there may be a proliferative form of the disease. Thrombosis of the arteriosclerotic anterior descending branch of the left coronary artery produces an infarct in the apex of the anterior wall of the left ventricle. Thrombosis of the circumflex branch of the left coronary artery produces infarction of the remainder of the heart. Thrombosis of the posterior descending branch of the right coronary artery produces infarction in the posterior wall of the left ventricle and adjacent portion of the right ventricle.

Inflammatory Diseases of Arteries. *Arteritis* is an inflammation of arteries due to local inflammation which expands to involve the adjacent arteries. Primary forms of arteritis produce either local or general arterial disease. *Polyarteritis nodosa* or *periarteritis nodosa* is an inflammatory disease of medium-sized and small arteries. The disease primarily affects the visceral blood vessels and occurs as part of a hypersensitivity reaction.

Buerger's disease or thromboangitis obliterans is a rare disorder producing damage to peripheral arteries of the extremities. The etiology of Buerger's disease is obscure; however, it may be due to a hypersensitivity reaction in young adult males. The disease is present in individuals who smoke. Inflammation occurs in the walls of the arteries and veins with thrombosis of both arteries and veins. Recanalization takes place in the thrombotic arteries and veins.

Syphilitic arteritis is due to a primary inflammatory process located in the adventitia or media. Syphilis produces a perivascular inflammation which extends from the *vaso vasorum* to the media but not to the intima.

Cardiovascular Syphilis. The heart and aorta show alterations during cardiovascular syphilis. The ascending aorta is dilated and vertical grooves or bark-like areas are present on the intimal surface. The bark-like structures in the intima of the aorta are pathognomonic of syphilis. Aneurysms of the aorta are a complication of syphilitic aortitis. Involvement of the aortic valve is also pathognomonic for syphilis. Syphilis produces a widening or separation of the commissures of the aortic valve. Insufficiency of the aortic valve occurs in syphilis due to arteriosclerosis. The heart is hypertrophied in cardiovascular syphilis.

Aneurysms. An aneurysm is a localized dilatation of the arterial wall. The dilatation results from a weakened, damaged or necrotic arterial wall. Aneurysms of the large arteries only may occur in cardiovascular syphilis and are termed *syphilitic aneurysms.* An infected embolus may cause necrosis of the media of arteries resulting in an aneurysm. The latter type of lesion is termed a *mycotic aneurysm.* In a true aneurysm the outpouching or sac is formed by the adjacent tissue. A *fusiform aneurysm* is a dilatation of a section of a vessel and occurs in the aorta and its larger branches. A *dissecting aneurysm* does not fulfill the requirements of a true aneurysm. Hemorrhage takes place into the media of the aorta and the hemorrhage dissects the vessel wall into two distinct layers.

DISEASES OF VEINS

Varicose Veins. Dilated, tortuous thick-walled peripheral veins are termed *varicose veins.* Varicose veins are commonly located in the lower extremities of individuals who stand on their feet while performing their duties. Women who have borne children are also prone to develop varicose veins. Hemorrhage may occur from varicose veins located in the esophagus. Hemorrhoids are a local form of varicose veins.

Phlebitis. Phlebitis is an inflammation resulting from an extension of a local infection which involves the walls of the veins. The infected vein may be the site of thrombosis. The latter events lead to *thrombophlebitis.* The inflammation in the wall of the vein may be low grade and the thrombosis firmly attached so that pulmonary embolism is not common. A highly virulent infection may be responsible for septic emboli in the pulmonary vessels and lung abscesses.

Phlebothrombosis. When blood coagulates intravenously in normal veins following heart failure, pregnancy, or compression of veins by neoplasms, the situation is termed *phlebothrombosis.* One-half percent of obstetrical patients develop phlebothrombosis. One percent of all major surgical patients develop phlebothrombosis. The veins generally develop thrombosis eight days following surgery. Blood circulates more slowly through the legs; therefore, the majority of postoperative thrombosis occurs in the veins of the leg. Because of the possibility of pulmonary embolism, patients do not remain in bed but generally walk on the first and second postoperative days.

DISEASES OF LYMPHATICS

Lymphangitis. Inflammation of the lymphatics is termed *lymphangitis.* Spread may occur from the inflamed lymphatics to the lymph nodes. Inflammation of the lymphatics appears as red streaks in the skin when the inflammation is superficial.

Lymphedema. An increase in tissue fluids resulting from obstruction of the lmyphatics of an area is termed *lymphedema.* Blockage of lymphatics occurs by neoplastic cells, and parasites in the lymphatics. The edema is localized to the tissues drained by the blocked lymphatics.

Chapter 12

DISEASES OF THE RESPIRATORY SYSTEM

PULMONARY EDEMA

When an obstruction occurs in the alveoli, the air pressure drops; therefore, edema occurs into the alveoli. Anoxia and damage to capillary walls, which take place during shock, are responsible for exudation of edema fluid into the alveoli. Left ventricular heart failure increases the hydrostatic pressure in the pulmonary capillaries and edema occurs in the alveoli. The latter is the most common cause of pulmonary edema. During pulmonary edema the alveolar walls are hyperemic and the alveolar spaces are filled with a pink-staining, homogeneous fluid. The fluid comprising edema of the lung consists of a rich protein fluid which is an excellent culture media for microorganisms.

Chronic passive hyperemia of the lung is due to right heart failure. The alveolar walls of the lung are thickened and macrophages containing hemosiderin (heart failure cells) are present in the alveoli. Although pulmonary emboli are uncommon, they may cause sudden death when an embolus occludes the pulmonary artery.

PULMONARY EMBOLISM AND INFARCTION

A 23-year-old pregnant female succumbed following delivery. At autopsy, an examination of the lungs revealed the presence of an amniotic fluid embolus. During labor, this pregnant female ruptured her membrane. Sudden contractions caused the amniotic fluid to enter a large open vein. The amniotic fluid embolus terminated in the lung producing a pulmonary infarction.

ATELECTASIS

Atelectasis is the collapse of a completely expanded lung. Primary atelectasis occurs physiologically in infants and newborns. Secondary atelectasis occurs in adults after a complete (not partial) bronchial obstruction. In an incomplete atelectasis, total collapse of the lung eventually occurs; however, it takes place late in the disease. Extrinsic fluid located in the chest may cause a collapse of the lung. A mechanical collapse of the lungs occurs by opening the chest. The primary atelectatic lung is airless, the lung tissue is not crepitant (crackling) or spongy. Secondary atelectasis consists of a collapsed lung containing black pigmentation (anthracosis).

INFECTIOUS DISEASES OF THE LUNGS

Three types of infectious diseases occur in the lungs, i.e. pulmonary abscesses and the bronchiectatic lung; bacterial pneumonias; and pulmonary infections due to higher forms of bacteria, fungi, viruses and parasites.

Bronchiectasis. Bronchiectasis is a term meaning the dilatation of bronchi of the lung. Two types of dilatations may occur in the bronchi, i.e. a local cystic or saccular dilated bronchus and a diffuse, fusiform or cylindrical dilated bronchus. Bronchiectasis may be congenital and appears at birth. Acquired bronchiectasis occurs as a result of infection and overdistention of one bronchus or of a group of bronchi due to a chronic bronchitis. Purulent exudate accumulates in the bronchi. The overdistention of the bronchi results from tearing of the elastic fibers in the bronchial wall. A neoplasm may cause partial obstruction to a bronchus. During inspiration a slight dilatation occurs in the bronchus as the air passes the partial obstruction. Complete obstruction develops during expiration. The air is trapped by the neoplasm which is obstructing the bronchi. Distal to the obstruction the lung shows emphysema, i.e. a pathologic increase in the air content of the lung, and the bronchi show bronchiectasis.

Pneumonitis. Beta-hemolytic streptococci, *Hemophilus influenza,* pneumococcus, and viruses provoke pneumonia. Beta-hemolytic streptococci and *Hemophilus influenza* cause interstitial pneumonia.

An anatomic classification of the pneumonias is the best available classification; however, this classification contains some deficiencies. The anatomic classification includes the following types of pneumonia: bronchopneumonia, lobar pneumonia, influenzal pneumonia, primary atypical pneumonia, interstitial pneumonia, and epidemic pneumonia of the newborn. Pneumonia generally begins as a tracheobronchitis accompanied by a dry cough. The infection extends into the alveolar walls and peribronchial tissue. The respiratory disease begins in the upper respiratory tract extending downward to the tracheobronchial tree.

Bronchopneumonia is an inflammation of the bronchi and peribronchial alveoli due to beta-hemolytic streptococcus in 3 to 5 percent; to staphylococcus in one percent; and to Friedlander's bacillus in one percent of infections of the lung. *Eschericia coli,* pneumococcus, *Hemophilus influenza* and *Nisseria catarrhalis* also produce pneumonia.

Pain is either absent or minimal during bronchopneumonia. The pleura is smooth and irregular nodularity occurs throughout the entire lung. Groups of peribronchial alveoli are affected by the infection and a purulent exudate is present in the bronchi and alveoli.

Lobar pneumonia involves an entire lobe or lobes of the lung, all consolidated as a unit in the same stage of pneumonitis. It is difficult to accurately separate the infection into definite stages; however, lobar pneumonia has four stages. Lobar pneumonia produces a pleuritis, and therefore pain in the chest is a common finding during the early stages of the infection.

TABLE XV

CLASSIFICATION OF PNEUMONIA

Anatomic Varieties of Pneumonia	Most Common Pathologic Organism	Gross Findings	Microscopic Findings
(1) Lobar (lobular form)	Diplococci, Pneumococci, Friedlander's bacilli, Streptococci	(1) inflammatory edema, dull gray-red lungs (2) early red hepatization (3) fibrinous gray hepatization (4) resolution	Dilated capillaries, edema PMN, fibrin, RBC Capillary engorgement Fibrinous material in alveoli Macrophages, fibrin dissolved
(2) Bronchopneumonia	Pneumococci, Streptococci, Staphylococci, Hemophilus influenzae Klebsella pneumoniae Friedlander's bacillus	Multiple focal or patchy lesions Example (1) lipid pneumonia, lipid in mononuclear cells (2) aspiration pneumonia	Groups of peribronchial alveoli are affected Purulent exudate is present in bronchi and peribronchial alveoli
(3) Interstitial pneumonia (interstitial bronchopneumonia)	Beta-hemolytic streptococcus, Virus, Hemophilus influenza	Complication is bronchiectasis Example (1) primary atypical pneumonia, (2) influenzae pneumonia, (3) epidemic pneumonia of newborn	Hemorrhagic bronchopneumonia Plasma cells, RBC and leukocytes, no fibrin Tracheobronchitis, Necrosis of walls of alveoli and thrombosis Few PMN leukocytes, Mononuclear response present
(4) Primary atypical pneumonia		Auto-hemagglutinins clamp red blood cells at 0°C. Related to antibody-like activity of acute phase serum (cold agglutins)	Inflammation in alveolar walls Alveoli are not involved
(5) Influenzal pneumonia			Necrosis of alveolar walls. Thrombosis of lymphatics and capillaries

Lobar pneumonia is due to pneumococci, types 1, 2 and 4; and diplococcus or pneumococcus in approximately 90 percent of instances of the infection. The infection spreads from the upper respiratory tract into the terminal bronchi. The organisms spread rapidly from the hilus to the periphery of the lung in a matter of hours. The infection spreads under the pleura causing an early pleuritis. The initial stage of lobar pneumonia is termed the *congestion stage*. The lung is red and congested or hyperemic. Edema and microorganisms are present in the alveoli along with a fibrinous exudate.

The second stage of lobar pneumonia is termed *red hepatization*. The alveolar walls are hyperemic and edema, blood, fibrin and polymorphonuclear leukocytes are present in the alveoli. Red hepatization produces a solid lung.

The third stage of lobar pneumonia is termed *gray hepatization*. Pneumococci, and fibrin are present; however, leukocytes disappear. Gray hepatization produces adherent lobes with loss of the normal lobar fissures of the lungs. The pleura is thickened during gray hepatization.

TABLE XVI

SYMPTOMS OF THE PNEUMONIAS

Bronchopneumonia

Not homogeneous.

No pain, no pleuritis, pleura smooth.

Irregular nodularity, groups of alveoli involved around central bronchus.

Pus from bronchi and alveoli.

Some areas normal, others involved.

Confluent bronchopneumonia—nodules fuse together.

Terminal bronchopneumonia is due to carcinoma.

Lobar Pneumonia

Homogeneous.

Pain, early pleuritis, pleura rough.

All areas involved equally in some stage of consolidation.

Infection travels through pores of Kohn.

Involves whole lobe or lobes.

Rapid spread of organisms from hilus to periphery under pleura.

Leads to early pleuritis.

Stages:

    (1) Congestion, hyperemia, edema (pneumococci in all alveoli)

    (2) Red hepatization $\longrightarrow$ pneumococci + RBC

    (3) Gray hepatization $\longrightarrow$ necrosis, hemolysis of RBC

    (4) Resolution $\longrightarrow$ lung becomes perfectly normal after resolution.

Lobular Pneumonia

Form of lobar pneumonia.

Involves lobules, not an entire lobe.

Newborn Viral Pneumonia

Cytomegalic inclusions in cells of bronchial epithelium.

Interstitial Mononuclear Reaction in Pneumonia

Involves alveolar walls as interstitial bronchopneumonia.

Severe tracheobronchitis (ulcerated mucosa).

Pus in lumen, walls of bronchus necrotic.

Complication—bronchiectasis.

The fourth stage of lobar pneumonia is termed *resolution*. All foreign material disappears from the alveoli. Resolution requires several weeks. Organization is a severe complication of lobar pneumonia. However, lobar pneumonia is rarely seen in modern times.

Another epidemic variety of pneumonia is termed *influenzal pneumonia*. In this variety of pneumonitis, the walls of the alveoli undergo necrosis with thrombosis of lymphatics and capillaries.

The clinical syndrome of *primary atypical pneumonia* includes a cough, cyanosis and a few rayles. However, the alveoli are not involved because the inflammation is localized to the alveolar walls. Cold agglutins are high in primary atypical pneumonia.

Interstitial pneumonia is a term describing the pathogenesis of bronchopneumonia. Epidemic interstitial bronchopneumonia is due to beta-hemolytic streptococci. The lungs are congested, and edematous with dilated bronchi.

Epidemic pneumonia of the newborn is a viral pneumonia. Cytomegalic viral inclusions are present in the cells of the bronchial epithelium. A thick hyaline membrane lines the alveoli in this viral pneumonia.

Lung Abscess. The formation of abscesses in the lung represents a serious infection because of the lack of resistance of pulmonary tissue. Lung abscesses develop secondarily to bacterial pneumonias and are also due to trauma, atelectasis and pleura effusions. Aerobic streptococci and staphylococci, and anaerobic fusobacterium, micrococci, streptococci, and bacteriodes are present in lung abscesses.

Hyaline Membrane Disease of Infancy. Hyaline membrane disease of infancy is a fatal disorder producing difficulty in breathing after birth so that retraction of the sternum takes place during inhalation. Obstruction occurs in the trachea and large or small bronchi. The child is cyanotic (blue) and anoxic.

Laboratory Diagnosis of the Pneumonias. Laboratory diagnosis of the pneumonias is made, in part, by sputum studies to determine the predominating organism responsible for the pneumonia. Fresh single sputum samples originating in the bronchi are utilized for laboratory diagnosis. A series of single specimens are necessary before a definitive diagnosis is established. Every twenty-four hours a sample of bronchial sputum is obtained for the sputum studies. The sputum is collected in a sterile wide-mouth bottle which is well stoppered to prevent contamination by other microorganisms. The sputum is cultured on blood agar. The aerobic organisms are further cultured on broth. Initially, a smear is prepared of the sputum in order to report the tentative diagnosis to the clinician. Within forty-five hours the microbiology laboratory will report the results of the cultured sputum reporting on the predominate organism. Microbiologic studies are useful in the acute stage of bronchiectasis because the microorganisms present may vary from aerobic to anaerobic types.

In pulmonary infections due to tubercle bacilli, three sputum examinations are generally undertaken and the smear is prepared using the acid fast stain. If the organisms on the smear prove to be tubercle bacilli, it still does not provide definite evidence that tuberculosis is present. The tubercle bacilli must first be cultured and then inoculated into guinea pigs. A period of three to eight weeks is required before the guinea pig develops the infection and succumbs to tuberculosis.

BRONCHIAL ASTHMA AND EMPHYSEMA

In bronchial asthma there is an increase in the secretion of mucous into the bronchi causing dilatation of the bronchial wall. A spasm in the bronchial wall traps air behind a partial obstruction created by the secretion of mucous and accompanying exudate. The obstruction may rupture alveoli and tear the elastic tissue present in the wall of alveoli. Overdistention of the lung may occur in asthma and result in emphysema. The emphysematous lung remains enlarged because the elastic tissue in the wall of alveoli is torn; therefore, the lung cannot collapse.

Emphysema results from chronic bronchitis, pulmonary tuberculosis, whooping cough and bronchial asthma. The following findings are considered pathognomonic of emphysema: decrease in alveolar depth, increase in alveolar diameter and flattening of alveolar bases.

PNEUMOCONIOSIS

Any foreign material, animate or inanimate, inhaled into the lungs causes a reaction in the lungs termed *pneumoconiosis*. Anthracosis is due to a foreign material which does not produce a true pneumoconiosis because no tissue reaction is elaborated by the body. Berylliosis is a true pneumoconiosis. Beryllium may be inhaled from either defective or broken florescent lights. A transitory pneumonitis results from the inhalation of beryllium. Asbestosis is a pneumoconiosis due to the inhalation of asbestos fibers. A high incidence of carcinoma of the lung appears to be associated with pneumoconiosis due to the inhalation of asbestos.

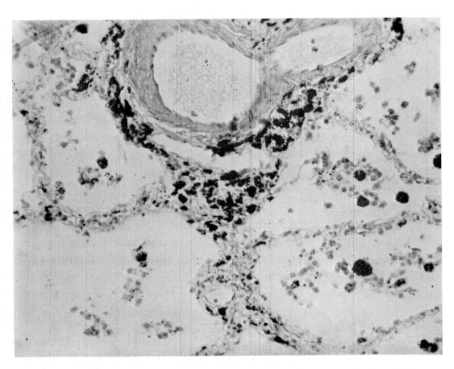

Figure 51. Anthracosis of the lung. Notice the carbon pigment in focal and linear type deposits within the alveolar walls. The alveolar phagocytes located in the lumen of the alveoli also contain carbon pigment.

Silicosis is the most important pneumoconiosis because silica is present in all minerals. Anthracosilicosis (miner's lung) is due to inhalation of coal and silica. The lung contains raised gray nodules, becomes solid, and no longer crepitant. Siderosilicosis is due to inhalation of iron and silica. Silicosis does not develop for approximately three to fifteen years following the initial inhalation of silica. Tuberculosis accounts for 75 percent of deaths in individuals with silicosis. An intense tissue reaction takes place around the silica particles consisting of a proliferation of connective tissue involving an intense proliferation of reticulum.

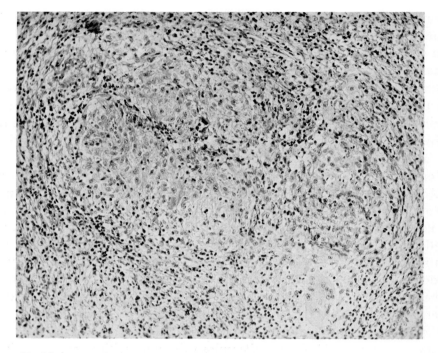

Figure 52. Blastomycosis of the lung. Notice the pulmonary lesion (tubercle) of blastomycosis which appears similar to tuberculosis. The tubercle of blastomycosis can be differentiated from tuberculosis by the presence of the blastomycetes organism and leukocytes in the lung tissue.

moniliasis. Monilia infection is found in the lungs of patients with any type of debilitating pulmonary disease.

Actinomycosis is a fungal disease which infects the lungs. *Actinomycosis bovis* is the most common member of this group and is capable of infecting the lung.

NEOPLASMS OF THE LUNG

Carcinoma of the lung is one of the most prevalent carcinomas in humans. Fifteen percent of all carcinomas in the human body are carcinomas of the lung. Lung carcinoma occurs between forty-five and sixty-five years of age. A higher instance of pulmonary carcinoma occurs in the right lung compared to the left lung primarily because the right lung is larger. Males have a higher incidence of carcinoma of the lung than females by a three to one ratio.

Factors to be considered in the production of lung carcinoma include the following carcinogens: (1) arsenic is a carcinogenic agent and is present in cigarette papers, (2) hydrocarbons in the smoke are carcinogens, (3) radium produces a high incidence of lung carcinoma, and (4) asbestos is associated with a high incidence of lung carcinoma.

The initial signs and symptoms of carcinoma of the lung include the following: atypical pneumonitis, atelectasis and bronchiectasis, cough, dyspnea, pain, and enlarged bronchial lymph nodes. The first sign of lung carcinoma may be the presence of hepatic and cerebral metastases. Carcinoma of the lungs is the most widely metastasizing of all carcinomas. Carcinomas of the lung are moderately radioresponsive.

Bronchial Adenoma. Bronchial adenomas represent the most important benign neoplasm of the bronchi and lung. Bronchial adenomas may undergo malignant transformation and metastasize to the regional lymph nodes. The mean age for the occurrence of bronchial adenomas is twenty-eight years.

Bronchogenic Carcinoma. Primary lung carcinoma is principally bronchogenic in origin and develops from the bronchial mucosa. There are three basic types of bronchogenic carcinomas of the lung, i.e. the *squamous cell carcinoma,* the *adenocarcinoma* and the *anaplastic carcinoma* (oat cell carcinoma).

Squamous cell carcinoma of the lung is the most common bronchogenic carcinoma. It represents 40 to 60 percent of all pulmonary carcinomas. Over 90 percent of squamous cell carcinomas of the lung occur in male cigarette smokers. There is strong evidence that lung carcinoma is due to heavy cigarette smoking. Squamous cell carcinoma generally arises from the bronchi adjacent to the hilus of the lung. Metastatic squamous cell carcinomas from the pharynx, larynx and oral cavity may metastasize to the lungs and therefore may be *readily confused* with primary bronchogenic carcinoma of the lungs. The development of the squamous cell carcinoma may be preceded by metaplasia of the cylindrical bronchial epithelium to squamous epithelium.

The adenocarcinoma is the rarest of the bronchogenic carcinomas. Thirty-five percent of bronchogenic carcinomas in females are adenocarcinomas. The adenocarcinoma may occur as an undifferentiated (anaplastic) bronchogenic carcinoma arising from the mucous secreting glands of the bronchi.

The anaplastic carcinoma or oat cell carcinoma arises from the bronchial epithelium of the main stem bronchi. It comprises approximately 40 percent of the bronchogenic carcinomas. The anaplastic carcinoma spreads by the lymphatics and blood stream. Metastases are present in approximately 90 percent of instances due to the explosive spread of neoplastic oat cells.

Bronchiolar carcinoma represents a fourth type of carcinoma of the lung. The bronchiolar carcinoma (alveolar cell carcinoma) develops from the cells of the terminal bronchioles or cells lining the alveoli of the lung. The bronchiolar carcinoma generally arises from the mucous secreting epithelium of the terminal bronchioles. Bronchiolar carcinoma represents less than 4 percent of all forms of lung carcinoma.

Bronchogenic carcinomas spread far and wide. Metastatic neoplasms may be the initial evidence that a primary carcinoma of the lung is present. Bronchogenic carcinomas spread throughout the lungs by way of the lymphatics and bronchioles. The neoplasm spreads to lymph nodes by way of the lymphatics and to distant organs by way of the blood stream and lymphatics.

Chapter 13

DISEASES OF THE GENITOURINARY SYSTEM

CONGENITAL ABNORMALITIES OF THE KIDNEYS

Agenesis of the Kidney. Renal agenesis may be unilateral or bilateral (incompatible with life). The newborn presents the following external features at birth which indicate agenesis of the kidneys: complete absence or diminished amniotic fluid, long and low placed ear lobes, receding chin, prominent intercantus of the eye, increased spacing between the eyes, and flattened tip of the nose.

Congenital Hypoplasia and Dysplasia of the Kidney. The true hypoplastic kidney is a small organ regardless of the age of the individual. In the hypoplastic kidney a reduction is present in both the nephrons and glomeruli. Unilateral hypoplasia is more common than the bilateral form. If one kidney is not functioning, the other kidney becomes enlarged due to compensatory hypertrophy.

Abnormality of position may result in the fusion of two kidneys producing the horseshoe kidney. In the horseshoe kidney an isthmus is present in the caudal portion joining the two kidneys. The kidney may migrate and become fused with the kidney on the opposite side forming either a double kidney or a fused single kidney. Ectopic kidneys occur when they move downward from their normal site.

Congenital polycystic disease of the kidney is generally bilateral; rarely is it unilateral. Congenital polycystic kidney is divided into two types, i.e. the congenital infantile and the congenital adult types. The congenital infantile polycystic kidney is initiated *in utero* and undergoes a prenatal increase in size so that the combined weight of the kidneys is 600 gm. The fetus lives *in utero* with the polycystic kidney because it is not dependent on renal filtration. However, the newborn may succumb several days or weeks following delivery due to renal failure. Cysts may occupy the majority of the renal substance, therefore only a few nephrons are left to operate. Adult congenital polycystic disease of the kidney begins *in utero* and is found in late infancy, childhood, young adults and adults from forty to sixty years of age. The disease is present throughout the life of the individual.

DISEASES OF THE KIDNEYS WHICH TERMINATE IN UREMIA

Uremia. Uremia is of unknown etiology and represents the terminal phase of renal insufficiency. Uremia is due to the retention of metabolic nitrogenous products which are generally excreted by the kidney. The complex findings consist of the following: acidosis, high concentration of urea, nitrogen, uric acid, and acid creatinine in the blood. The calcium/phosphorus ratio is abnormal with a great increase in phosphorus and decrease in calcium. The kidneys are unable to concentrate urine or to function under increased demands. Uremia may be accompanied by bone changes and hypoplasia of the parathyroid glands, *uremic pericarditis,* edematous lungs, edematous brain, gastrointestinal tract hemorrhage, necrosis of the spleen termed *spotted spleen,* inspissation of secretions in the pancreas, and hemorrhages in the skin and mucous membranes. A frost forms over the skin termed *uremic frost.*

The tissue alterations in uremia due to renal failure start in the glomeruli as a glomerulonephritis. Renal failure is preceded by vascular lesions which cause destruction of glomeruli and nephrons, and by bacterial infection and inflammation which destroys the glomeruli.

Glomerulonephritis. Glomerulonephritis is an inflammation of the glomerular tufts. The inflammation may result in proliferation or exudation in the glomeruli. The etiology of the disease is obscure; however, it is related to infection probably with streptococci. The disease may be the result of an allergic phenomena of renal tissue to microorganisms or their products. There are three stages of glomerulonephritis, i.e. acute, subacute and chronic. The three stages are not distinct entities but rather blend together into one disease entity.

Acute glomerulonephritis may be initiated by group A hemolytic streptococcus—type 12 in young individuals. The surface of the kidneys is smooth and is studded with numerous petechial hemorrhages (flea-bitten kidney). The enlarged glomeruli are highly cellular due to the proliferation of capillary endothelium, exudation of polymorphonuclear leukocytes in the glomerular tufts and thrombi in the capillaries. The flow of blood through the glomeruli is slowed resulting in decreased output of urine, and leakage of red blood cells and albumin into the urine. Diffuse involvement of glomeruli during acute glomerulonephritis may result in death.

Subacute glomerulonephritis may be accompanied by uremia in a matter of months. The kidneys are enlarged, mottled yellow, and there is involvement of practically all of the glomeruli. The most prominent alteration in the glomeruli consists of proliferation of the epithelium of the capsule of the glomeruli to form "glomerular crescents." The glomerular tufts are, however, separated from the glomerular crescents and hyalinized tufts are generally absent. The tubules become atrophic and contain red cell casts. The urinary output is normal or decreased and large amounts of protein are excreted in the urine. The plasma proteins are diminished and A/G ratio is reversed to 1/1. Subacute glomerulonephritis may be unilateral; however, this phase is generally a bilateral diffuse form of the disease.

Chronic glomerulonephritis may follow the acute and subacute forms of the disease by a progressive failure of renal function. The disease slowly

TABLE XVIII

CLINICAL AND LABORATORY FINDINGS IN GLOMERULONEPHRITIS

Acute Glomerulonephritis

Increased urine
Red blood cells in urine
Few casts in urine
Albuminuria
Minor tubular changes
Latent period
Elevated blood pressure
Enlarged kidney
Mottled red external surface of kidney due to hemorrhage
Capsule of kidney not adherent
Forms of acute glomerulonephritis
  Hemorrhagic
  Exudative
  Thrombotic (necrotizing)
  Proliferative

Subacute Glomerulonephritis

Formation of crescents
Anasarca
Normal or diminished Urine
Albuminuria
Decreased plasma proteins
Reversal of A/G ratio (1:1 instead of 2:1)
Hypercholesterolemia
Hypoproteinemia
Elevated blood pressure
Capsule of kidney not adherent
Enlarged kidney

Chronic Glomerulonephritis

Elevated nitrogen in blood
Hypertension
Minimal edema
Increased urinary output and nocturia
Decreased albuminuria
Hyperproteinemia
Casts in urine
Specific gravity of urine 1.012 (maximum level)
Contracted small kidney
Adherent capsule of kidney
Irregular granular surface of kidney

progresses for many years with minimal clinical symptoms. However, there is a decrease of renal function. The terminal phase of the disease is always the development of uremia and an inability to concentrate urine. The unconcentrated urine is therefore excreted in large quantities producing nocturia and polyuria.

Grossly, depressed zones are present on the surface of the kidney. These zones represent scars located beneath the capsule. The elevated portion of the surface of the kidney represents areas of viable nephrons. The kidneys are small and contracted during chronic glomerulonephritis.

Numerous glomeruli are converted into partial hyaline areas or a complete hyalinization takes place in the capillary tufts. The renal tubules undergo atrophic changes and there is an increase in the interstitial connective tissue around the glomeruli and between the tubules. The tubules contain hyaline casts. Some glomeruli show capsular adhesions and are highly cellular. Hypertension develops in the terminal phase of chronic glomerulonephritis as a result of loss of the glomerular nephrons, scarring, and vascular

TABLE XIX

ETIOLOGY OF CONTRACTED AND FLEA-BITTEN KIDNEY

Cause of the Contracted Kidney
> Chronic glomerulonephritis
> Chronic arteriolar nephrosclerosis
> Malignant hypertension
> Chronic pyelonephritis

Causes of the Flea-bitten Kidney
> Acute glomerulonephritis
> Embolic glomerulonephritis
> Early malignant nephrosclerosis (essential hypertension)

TABLE XX

MANIFESTATIONS AND ETIOLOGY OF UREMIA

Manifestations of Uremia
> Azotemia
> Urineferous oral odor
> Disturbance of water balance
> Disturbance of electrolyte balance (loss of sodium,
>   retention of potassium)
> Disturbance in regulation of acid-base balance
> Diarrhea and lesions in gastrointestinal tract
> Eye ground changes and hypertension

Causes of Uremia
> Chronic glomerulonephritis
> Chronic pyelonephritis
> Lower nephron nephrosis
> Acute tubular necrosis
> Arteriolar nephrosclerosis (malignant hypertension)

sclerosis. It may be difficult to distinguish between nephrosclerosis and chronic glomerulonephritis. A secondarily contracted kidney indicates that it has passed through the stages of acute and subacute glomerulonephritis.

VASCULAR DISEASE OF THE KIDNEY

Thrombosis of the renal artery, arteriosclerosis, and renal venous thrombosis may result in infarction of the kidney. Changes in the small vessels of the kidney are almost invariably associated with an elevated blood pressure.

Glomerulonephritis is associated with hypertension. A small change is readily produced in the vessels of the kidney during hypertension. Diffuse changes occur in the arterioles throughout the body as well as in the kidney during hypertension. Essential hypertension occurs when the systolic pressure is over 200 and the diastolic pressure is 130. Alterations in the nephrons are due to narrowing of the interlobular artery which results from atrophic changes. Glomeruli shrink into hyalinized balls due to a deficient blood supply to the glomeruli. Nephrons in the area undergo atrophic changes. However, not all nephrons undergo hyalinization and some nephrons are retained in a normal state. The contracted kidney does not have a normal blood supply and is poorly vascularized. It is possible for some nephrons to survive because they obtain blood by means of anastomosis. Grossly, due to essential hypertension the contracted kidney has an adherent capsule and a granular surface.

Essential hypertension is due to nephrosclerosis, fibrosis and the contracted kidney. Seven to ten percent of individuals with essential hypertension die of uremia. Essential hypertension may be complicated by malignant hypertension. Malignant nephrosclerosis may be superimposed on early or late essential hypertension.

Malignant nephrosclerosis produces alterations in arterioles termed *necrotizing arteriolitis*. The necrotizing change is superimposed on hyaline arteriolar changes which occur in the less affected arterioles. No structures are recognized in malignant nephrosclerosis. The afferent arterioles, glomeruli and capillary tufts undergo fibrinoid necrosis. In malignant nephrosclerosis the patient generally dies of uremia and cardiovascular changes.

PYELONEPHRITIS

Pyelonephritis is another renal disease leading to a contracted kidney. Glomerulonephritis, arteriolar nephrosclerosis, malignant nephrosclerosis and pyelonephritis all terminate in the contracted kidney and uremia. The hypertension which accompanies unilateral pyelonephritis is curable. However, the hypertension which accompanies bilateral pyelonephritis in incurable. Enterococci, *Proteus vulgaris, Escherichia coli, Pseudomonas aeruginosa* and *Aerobacter aerogenes* are responsible for the development of pyelonephritis. The disease generally reaches the kidneys by the ascending route and is commonly due to an obstructive phenomenon causing stasis of fluid. In pyelonephritis the infection may be of the uncommon descending type in which instance it spreads downward to involve the kidney.

Grossly, the pyelonephritic kidney is enlarged with multiple abscesses located on the surface of the organ. Perinephritic abscesses occur since the infection spreads through the adherent capsule to the perirenal tissue. The individual may die of a suppurative pyelonephritis with renal failure, uremia, and sepsis. The pyelonephritis may, however, subside or undergo acute exacerbations.

In the chronic stages of pyelonephritis the kidney becomes small and contracted weighing approximately 100 gm. The surface contains irregular retracted areas with either smooth or granular parenchyma.

The kidney in acute glomerulonephritis is large, red and hemorrhagic. In subacute glomerulonephritis the kidney is large and pale. In chronic glomerulonephritis the kidney is small, pale and granular representing a secondary contracted kidney. In arteriolonephrosclerosis a red contracted kidney is present containing finely uniform granularity. In chronic pyelonephritis the kidney is contracted, irregularly scarred and granular.

TUBERCULOSIS OF THE KIDNEY

Tuberculosis of the kidneys may be unilateral or bilateral. The initial tubercular focus spreads to the calyces, infundibulum, pelvis and ureters. Tuberculosis of the mucous membrane of the pelvis has the gross appearance of a nonspecific ulcer. The infection starts in the renal pelvis which initially undergoes enlargement. Tubercle bacilli spread into a static urine and the bacilli ascend into the kidney proper resulting in infection of renal substance. Tubercles are studded irregularly over the surface of the thickened ureter and occur irregularly and conglomerantly throughout the substance of the kidney.

In tuberculous pyelonephritis the ureteral stricture is involved by ulceration, dilatation occurs in the pelvis, and the calyces are ulcerated. Two factors are responsible for enlargement of the pelvis and calyces, i.e. obstruction and retention of urine, and the progress of tuberculous ulcers with erosion of pyramids. If obstruction of the ureter occurs, the rate of progression of the tuberculosis is enhanced. The entire kidney may be replaced by caseation necrosis leaving a shell of viable renal tissue.

HYDRONEPHROSIS

Nephritis means inflammation of the kidney. Nephrosis means a degenerative change in the kidney. Hydronephrosis means a dilated renal pelvis and dilated infundibulum and calyces accompanied by degeneration of renal parenchyma due to pressure atrophy. Hydronephrosis is brought about either by a disturbance in the flow of urine from the renal pelvis or by a congenital abnormal nerve supply to the ureter.

In hydronephrosis the obstructive phenomenon produces a dilatation of the ureters and the renal pelvis. The pelvis enlarges as a result of the obstruction and hydronephrosis develops. A stricture may occur at the ureter-pelvic junction or stones may be present giving rise to hydronephrosis in the proximal or distal ureter. In hydronephrosis the pelvis and infundibulum are enlarged and the calyces become hollowed out. Hydronephrosis may occur accompanied by an acute infection of the kidney. The fluid which is present in hydronephrosis has a clear watery consistency. When suppuration is superimposed upon the hydronephrosis the clear fluid changes its character and a pyelonephrosis results, i.e. pyelonephritis plus hydronephrosis.

Expansion of the kidney and atrophy of the renal parenchyma occur in pyelonephrosis. The kidney increases from three to five times its normal size during hydronephrosis.

Renal calculi are renal stones which form in the kidney and may be found in the bladder. The calculi may be small in size and therefore are capable of migrating down the ureter resulting in ureteral cholic. The smaller calculi are generally passed by the patient. A spasm may occur in the ureter containing the renal calculi with resultant pain. Hydronephrosis may occur as a consequence or complication of the renal calculi. Large calculi occur in the renal pelvis and have the morphology of finger-like projections termed *staghorn renal calculi.*

NEOPLASMS OF THE KIDNEY

Benign Neoplasms of the Kidney. Benign neoplasms are frequently located in the kidney. *Fibromas* occur as nodules in the pyramids of the kidney. Occasionally smooth muscle combines with a fibrous connective tissue proliferation to form a *leiomyofibroma* of the kidney. Small *lipomas* are located in the cortex more frequently than in the medulla. *Leiomyomas* may occur in the renal parenchyma not associated with the fibroma. *Adenomas* occur in the scarred areas of the kidney as small well-circumscribed masses.

Papillomas occur in the renal pelvis and resemble papillomas of the bladder. The papilloma of the bladder has certain inherent dangers. The papilloma of the renal pelvis may have a benign architecture and still tend to spread down the ureter. The pelvic papilloma may become a frankly invasive neoplasm.

Malignant Neoplasms of the Kidney. *Wilms' tumor* is a rare neoplasm of the kidney in children, generally prior to seven years of age. Wilms' tumor is responsible for one-fifth of all of the malignant neoplasms of children. This neoplasm is a mixed tumor containing glandular elements and sarcomatous tissue both arising from misplaced mesodermal tissue which retains the ability to form both epithelial and connective tissues. Wilms' tumor grows rapidly, invades the surrounding tissue, and metastasizes by way of the blood stream to the brain, lymph nodes and liver.

Hypernephroma or renal cell carcinoma is a common malignant tumor of the kidneys of adults. Small foci of adrenal cells may be displaced to the kidney. It is hypothesized that the latter adrenal cells give rise to the hypernephroma. However, the latter observation is inconclusive and the hypernephroma is fundamentally an adenocarcinoma of the kidney which develops more frequently in males over forty years of age. This neoplasm consists of large clear cells in sheets and cords with minimal connective tissue stroma. The neoplasm grows causing atrophy of the kidney. In advanced stages there is widespread invasion of renal tissue. Metastases follow renal invasion to the bones, liver and lungs. The early stage of this neoplasm may be difficult to diagnose because clinical symptoms are minimal.

PELVIS AND URETER

Abnormalities of the Pelvis and Ureter. A double pelvis or two ureters are examples of abnormalities arising in the pelvis and ureters. The ureters either unite and fuse into a single structure, or they have separate openings into the bladder.

Ureteritis and Pyelitis. Inflammation of a ureter is termed *ureteritis* and inflammation of the pelvis of the kidney is termed *pyelitis*. Calculi may be associated with both ureteritis and pyelitis.

Neoplasms of the Pelvis and Ureter. Papillomas of the pelvis and ureter are benign neoplasms; however, they show a great tendency to recur. Malignant neoplasms of the pelvis and ureter include the papillary carcinoma, transitional cell carcinoma, and infiltrating squamous cell carcinoma.

URINARY BLADDER

Inflammatory Cystitis. Inflammation of the urinary bladder is termed *cystitis*. Inflammatory cystitis is generally secondary to infection in the surrounding organs and tissues and may follow the placement of a catheter or use of the cystoscope. The inflammation causes increased urination accompanied by burning and painful micturition. The urine contains pus, bacteria and albumin.

Neoplasms of the Urinary Bladder. *Benign neoplasms* (rare) of the urinary bladder have a tendency to recur following excision. The transitional papilloma is a histopathologically benign lesion which recurs and is considered a grade one transitional cell carcinoma. The *malignant neoplasms* of the urinary bladder include the *papillary transitional cell carcinoma, epidermoid carcinoma* and the *adenocarcinoma*. Papillary carcinoma is the most common neoplasm of epithelial origin occurring in the bladder. Hematuria, dysuria and secondary infection are clinical and are laboratory findings associated with papillary carcinoma of the urinary bladder. Epidermoid carcinoma is less common than the papillary carcinoma.

Chapter 14

DISEASES OF THE GASTROINTESTINAL TRACT

DISEASES OF THE ESOPHAGUS

Congenital Anomalies. Agenesis is complete absence or imperfect development of the esophagus. In atresia the upper portion of the esophagus ends blindly.

Diverticuli (acquired) may occur in the esophagus. In older individuals the diverticuli may become very large and contain a volume of 300 cc of fluid. If the mouth of the diverticulum is small, infection will result due to stagnation and a diverticulitis occurs. Diverticulitis may lead to perforation.

Circulatory Disturbances of the Esophagus. Submucosal and subserosal esophageal varices are due to distention of blood vessels. The esophageal varices may rupture with hemorrhage occurring from the point of rupture. Clinically the diagnosis of esophageal varices is made by utilizing balloons.

In cardiac patients or terminally in patients with debilitated disease a poor circulation occurs in the esophagus and an acute esophagitis with or without esophagomalacia (soft esophagus) develops.

Infections of the Esophagus. Infections of the esophagus are not common. Esophagitis may be due to monilia infection in infants. Acute and subacute esophagitis produces erosion and inflammation in the esophageal wall with desquamation of epithelial cells.

Scleroderma of the Esophagus. Scleroderma results in a firm, immovable (stiff) esophagus due to collagen degeneration in the wall.

Plummer-Vinson Syndrome. This syndrome produces the following symptoms in females between forty and fifty years of age: dysphagia, soreness and atrophy of the esophageal mucosa, achlorhydria, and hypochromic anemia. The dysphagia is caused either by a thin membranous web passing across the lumen of the esophagus or by narrow constricting bands which encircle the lumen of the esophagus. It has been hypothesized that the neoplasia associated with Plummer-Vinson syndrome arises in the atrophic esophageal mucosa.

Neoplasms of the Esophagus. Malignant neoplasms occur in the esophagus. The esophageal carcinoma is the only common neoplasm. It develops in males over fifty years of age. Fifty percent of esophageal carcinomas develop in the middle third of the esophagus, twenty-five percent in the lower third and twenty-five percent in the upper third. The squamous cell carcinoma is the predominant esophageal carcinoma. It invades the adjacent tissues and metastizes to the lymph nodes, liver and lungs.

DISEASES OF THE STOMACH

Anomalies of the Stomach. Gastric malrotation accompanied by intestinal malrotation is an anomaly occurring in the stomach. Diverticuli may be present in the fundus of the stomach. Atresia of the pylorus or cardiac regions of the stomach is a rare anomaly. Diaphragmatic hernia is the most common hernia which occurs in the chest.

Circulatory Disturbances of the Stomach. Circulatory disturbances occur in the stomach during congestive heart failure, due to focal obstruction, congestion of the stomach and terminally in cardiac patients. Gastromalacia may occur terminally in cardiac patients.

Inflammatory Lesions of the Stomach. *Acute gastritis* is an inflammation of the stomach caused by irritating substances, foods, alcohol and the ingestion of poisons. Prior to the advent of the antibiotics, a purulent gastritis (acute) occurred secondary to osteomyelitis, pneumonia and scarlet fever.

Chronic gastritis occurs in atrophic and hypertrophic forms. Chronic atrophic gastritis occurs during vitamin D deficiency, pernicious anemia, chronic alcoholism and chronic pellagra. The lining of the stomach contains flattened rugae and there is a reduction in the surface area of the gastric mucosa. The mucosal glands are decreased in number and leukocytes infiltrate the mucosa and submucosa. Metaplasia may occur in the gastric mucosa during chronic gastritis. The metaplasia is commonly present during carcinoma of the stomach. However, it has not been established whether the gastric metaplasia leads to the development of gastric carcinoma.

Chronic hypertrophic gastritis produces a lining mucosa which contains large rugae and a hypertrophic polypoid lining. The gastric mucosa is hyperplastic and lymphocytes and eosinophiles are infiltrated throughout the lamina propria.

Peptic Ulcer of the Stomach. Peptic ulcer is an erosion of the stomach because the gastric mucosa is a tissue that may be acted upon by acidic gastric juice. Acute peptic ulcers are small common superficial erosions produced by injuries (hot foods, coarse foods), blood stream infections, and skin burns. They generally heal rapidly in the gastric mucosa but occasionally may become chronic peptic ulcers.

Chronic peptic ulcers of the stomach are more common in males and Caucasians. Chronic peptic ulcers occur only in areas of the gastric mucosa which are exposed to the acidic gastric juice. Excessive acidity is commonly associated with the peptic ulcer of the stomach.

A circulatory theory for formation of the peptic ulcer states that an alteration occurs in the vascular supply of the gastric mucosa as a result of thrombosis. Local infections may produce the peptic ulcer. The neurogenic theory states that disturbances in the nervous system provoke the peptic ulcer. The gastric peptic ulcer generally develops proximal to the pyloric ring and in the pyloric portion of the stomach (posterior wall near lesser curvature). The gastric peptic ulcer is a single small ulcer which remains small. Chronic peptic ulcers of the stomach are punched-out indurated areas with hyperemia surrounding the ulcerations. The ulcer involves the mucosa, submucosa and muscular layers. The base of the ulcer consists of fibrous tissue and over the fibrous base are granulation tissue, necrotic tissue and an exudate of inflammatory cells. Healing of the peptic ulcer occurs by organization and fibrosis. The gastric mucosa grows over the fibrosis from the edges of the ulcer. Malignant transformation may occur in the chronic gastric peptic ulcer in less than five percent of peptic ulcerations.

Neoplasms of the Stomach. Benign neoplasms are not common and are of minor clinical significance. The common benign neoplasms of the stomach are the fibroma, lipoma, leiomyoma, gastric adenomatous polyps, and neurofibroma. The gastric mucosa may be the site of development of a single polypoid adenoma or of multiple polyps. The adenomatous polyps may rarely undergo malignant transformation.

The adenocarcinoma of the stomach is the most common and significant gastric malignant neoplasm. Gastric malignant neoplasms are responsible for approximately 10 percent of all deaths from neoplasia in the United States. Gastric carcinoma is more common in males after fifty years of age. Gastric carcinoma has a high incidence in Icelanders and Japanese. This neoplasm appears to have an hereditary susceptibility. Gastric adenocarcinoma may develop at any site in the stomach but more commonly arises from glandular cells located in the lesser curvature.

The adenocarcinoma of the stomach arises from the glandular and mucous cells of the stomach. The adenocarcinoma of the stomach appears as a large polypoid or cauliflower mass which extends into the lumen of the stomach. The adenocarcinoma spreads by direct expansion and invasion of adjacent and surrounding tissues as well as by the lymphatics and blood vessels. Gastric carcinomas metastasize to the liver, lungs, bones and regional lymph nodes.

Sarcomas represent only a small number of malignancies of the stomach. The lymphosarcoma, leiomyosarcoma and fibrosarcoma may rarely develop in the stomach.

DISEASES OF THE SMALL INTESTINES

Congenital Anomalies. The order of frequency of congenital anomalies is greatest in the duodenum, followed by the ileum, colon and jejunum. The duodenum, ileum, jejunum and colon may be the site of either *congenital atresia* or *stenosis*. Atresia is the closing down of the lumen of the bowel.

Meckel's diverticulum is an outgrowth or outpouching of the intestines located in the left abdomen and has been referred to as left-sided appendicitis. Meckel's diverticulum may become infected with the development of an acute Meckel's diverticulitis. Thirty percent of individuals with diverticuli in the small bowel show the presence of heterotrophic gastric mucosa which may cause a peptic ulcer complication. Meckel's diverticulum may, therefore, be the site of a bleeding peptic ulcer.

Vascular Disturbances. *Hyperemia, edema* and *hemorrhage* may occur in the small intestines. *Infarction* of the small intestines is due to occlusion of the superior or inferior mesenteric arteries by emboli or thrombi. The extent of an infarction of the small intestines is directly related to the size of the occluded vessel. The bowel proximal to the infarction becomes distended due to ileus. *Chronic passive congestion* of the small bowel occurs in males more commonly than females (3 to 2 ratio). This vascular disturbance has a sudden onset with acute paroxysmal abdominal pain. Chronic passive congestion of the small intestines is rarely localized and may be associated with reflex vomiting.

Inflammation. *Duodenal peptic ulcer* is a chronic peptic ulcer of the duodenum and probably has a similar etiology as the peptic ulcer located in the stomach and esophagus. Duodenal stasis, related to mesenteric occlusion at the duodenal-jejunal junction, may play a role in the etiology and pathogenesis of the duodenal peptic ulcer. The duodenal peptic ulcer is characterized clinically by pain, vomiting and hematemesis. The duodenal peptic ulcer may perforate, bleed, undergo scarring and produce stenosis. The ratio of gastric to duodenal peptic ulcer is 1:2 respectively. The duodenal peptic ulcer occurs most frequently between the ages of twenty and fifty years. Seventy-five percent of duodenal peptic ulcers occur in males. The duodenal peptic ulcer is generally located 2 to 3 cm below the pylorus along the posterior wall of the duodenum or lesser turn against the head of the pancreas. Microscopically, the duodenal peptic ulcer exhibits the following layers: the layer of exudation, the layer of necrosis, layer of granulation tissue, and the layer of scarring. An acute perforation (complication) may lead to generalized peritonitis. Massive hemorrhage or slow bleeding and stenosis are complications of the duodenal peptic ulcer.

Regional ileitis is an acute or chronic inflammatory disease of the bowel of obscure etiology. The inflammation occurs in the ileum in 60 percent of affected individuals, in the ileum and colon in 35 percent, and in the jejunum in 3.5 percent of the instances of regional ileitis. The disease is characterized by inflammation of all layers of the wall of the bowel. Clinical features include pain and formation of a mass or swelling.

A diffuse or circumscribed inflammation is evident accompanied by hyperplasia, hypertrophy and granular polypoid proliferation. Multiple ulcerations, perienteritis and pericolitis, stenosis, chronic perforation, fistula, peritonitis, thickened mesentery, and a tumor-like mass are associated with regional ileitis.

Intestinal Obstruction. Obstruction of the intestines indicates that a disturbance is present involving the intestinal contents which prevents their movement onward through the bowel lumen. Actual physical closure of the lumen, i.e. dynamic ileus, may be responsible for the obstruction. A disturbance may be present in muscular contraction resulting in cessation of intestinal motor activity, i.e. paralytic ileus.

The pathologic effects of intestinal obstruction are fluid and electrolyte loss, distention, changes in the wall of the bowel, absorption from obstructed bowel, strangulation, and mechanisms by which the obstruction causes death. Obstructions of the bowel may develop at a high or low level. If the obstruction is high, vomiting and loss of hydrochloric acid result. If the obstruction is low, abdominal distention and acidosis result.

Neoplasms of the Small Intestines. Benign neoplasms are rare in the small intestines. The lipoma, fibroma, leiomyoma and benign polyps may involve the small intestines. Carcinoma of the small intestines is rare. Malignancies of the small bowel are more common in males between fifty and sixty years of age. Adenocarcinoma causes obstruction and jaundice.

DISEASES OF THE APPENDIX

Congenital Anomalies. The congenital anomalies of the appendix include atresia, absence, reduplication and diverticulae.

Inflammatory Disease. *Acute appendicitis* is the most common disease of the abdomen necessitating surgical intervention. Appendicitis occurs equally in males and females. Fifty percent of instances of appendicitis occur in individuals under twenty years of age. The inflammation is rare in children. Appendicitis occurs in individuals living in highly civilized regions of the world. Clinically, the findings are abdominal pain, nausea, vomiting, leukocytosis, fever, rigidity at McBurney's point, and tenderness. Chronic appendicitis results from the acute inflammatory process. Fecaliths (stones) may cause stasis or obstruction in the distal one-third of the appendix. Foreign bodies are important factors in causing obstruction and appendiceal stasis. Lymphoid hyperplasia frequently occurs in teenagers and the resulting hyperplasia may obstruct the lumen of the appendix. Bacterial infection and obstruction are the two most important etiologic agents in the production of appendicitis.

Bacteriological investigations reveal that *Bacillus coli* was present in 57 percent, *Bacillus coli* and streptococci in 19 percent, and streptococci only in 9 percent of instances of appendicitis. Anaerobic microorganisms have been isolated in less than 50 percent, non-hemolytic streptococci and pneumococci in 100 percent, enterococci in 65 percent, gram positive rods and coliform group in 50 percent, gram negative rods of the influenzal form in 25 percent, and bacterium coli mucosum in 14 percent of instances of appendicitis.

The gross appearance of the appendix is dependent upon the type of inflammation, i.e. acute, suppurative, hemorrhagic, and gangrenous appendicitis. Histopathologically, the mucosa is edematous, hyperemic, and may be ulcerated. Polymorphonuclear leukocytes infiltrate the wall of the appendix.

Obliterative appendicitis occurs when the distal end of the lumen of the appendix is plugged by lymphoid tissue containing no mucosal covering. Chronic lymphoid appendicitis occurs in children and is usually accompanied by lymphadenitis.

Mucocele of the Appendix. Mucocele of the appendix occurs in the distal end. The mucocele of the appendix is due to obstruction. The lumen of the appendix becomes filled with mucin which arises from the glands of the mucosa and produces a morbidly distended appendix. Mucin fills the entire lumen of the appendix.

Carcinoid of the Appendix. Carcinoid (neoplasm) of the appendix commonly arises from theca cells located in the wall of the appendix. The benign carcinoid neoplasm initially involves the submucosa; however, it subsequently invades the remainder of the wall of the appendix.

DISEASES OF THE LARGE INTESTINES

Congenital Anomalies. *Anomalies of length and size,* i.e. *congenital megacolon or Hirschsprung disease* occurs in the large bowel. Megacolon means the presence of a markedly dilated descending or sigmoid colon. The marked intestinal dilatation is due to the congenital absence of neural elements in the segment of large bowel below the dilatation.

Diverticuli are common in the colon. Diverticuli develop in the weakened bowel wall at the site of entry of blood vessels. Herniation of the lining mucosa occurs into the wall of the colon and the muscle layer is pushed aside. Diverticuli are commonly located in the descending and sigmoid colon. Approximately 10 percent of the population over sixty years of age develop diverticuli. Left-sided acute appendicitis is actually acute diverticulitis.

Vascular Disturbances. Infarction, hemorrhage and hemorrhoids represent the major vascular disturbances in the colon.

Inflammatory Diseases. *Tuberculosis* of the intestines is the most common secondary lesion of this granulomatous disease. Intestinal tuberculosis occurs as a result of dissemination of pulmonary tuberculosis. The iliocecal region is the most common intestinal site for the development of tuberculosis.

Typhoid fever involves the terminal ileum. The lesions of typhoid fever are located in the iliocecal region of the intestines. The lymph nodes, spleen, liver and reticuloendothelial system are involved during typhoid fever. Swelling and congestion of Peyer's patches of the terminal ileum are the principal alterations. Stuffing and ulceration develop in the intestinal mucosa at the sites of Peyer's patches.

Bacillary dysentary produces lesions in the sigmoid colon and rectum. The intestinal lesion appears as a superficial ulceration with a pseudomembrane covering the ulceration.

Endamoebic dysentary involves the cecum and rectum. Minimal inflammation is present; however, small, superficial ulcerations develop in the mucosa of the cecum and rectum. Endamoeba histolyticus enters the wall of the cecum producing a deep flask-shaped ulceration.

Regional ileitis or enteritis is a disease of unknown origin. The disease may involve any portion of the ileum; however, the terminal portion of the ileum is most commonly involved. Approximately twenty to thirty centimeters of the terminal ileum are generally involved in regional ileitis. The alteration which occurs is well demarcated at both ends of the inflammatory zone. The gross lesion of an ileitis has the appearance of a carcinoma.

Ulcerative colitis is an inflammatory disease of the colon of obscure etiology. *Chronic ulcerative colitis* is a specific inflammatory disease of the colon occurring in middle adult life. Proposed etiologic factors are allergy, infection, neurogenic disturbances, and enzymatic necrosis of the colon. The disease is accompanied by remissions and exacerbations over an extended period of time. An edematous large intestine, rectum and sigmoid colon undergoes necrosis and ulceration. The ulcerations are small; however, coalescence of individual ulcerations may result in formation of large and very irregular ulcerations. The wall of the bowel undergoes fibrosis and thickening and the ulcerations undergo resolution by fibrosis and scarring. Perforation, hemorrhage and peritonitis are severe complications. Multiple polypoid masses may be associated with chronic ulcerative colitis.

Malignant transformation may occur in the polypoid proliferations associated with chronic ulcerative colitis. Carcinoma has a greater instance in the colon affected with chronic ulcerative colitis when compared to the unaffected colon.

Uremia causes superficial nonspecific ulcers in the colon.

Benign Neoplasms. Benign neoplasms are rare in the large bowel. Benign adenomas or adenomatous polyps develop in the colon as polypoid, sessile or ulcerated benign gross neoplasms. The adenomatous polyp may have a predisposition to undergo malignant change. However, this change is currently debatable. Multiple adenomas or benign polyposis of the colon and rectum is a definite premalignant lesion in the descending colon, sigmoid colon, and rectum. Polyposis of the colon and rectum may occur as a diffuse disease (polyposis) or as a solitary disease (polyposis). The solitary polyposis consists of a few adenomatous polyps whereas the diffuse polyposis consists of a large number of polyps throughout the entire colon and rectum.

Malignant Neoplasms. Carcinoma of the large intestines is a very important neoplasm. Ninety-five percent of all malignant neoplasms of the intestines occur in the colon. One percent of all carcinomas (human) occur in the colon. Carcinoma of the large intestines is more common in males than females. It is rare in individuals under forty years of age. Fifty percent of carcinomas of the colon occur in the recto-sigmoid region. Two-thirds occur in the left colon and one-third in the right colon. Twenty-five percent of carcinomas of the large intestines occur in the sigmoid colon. Two predisposing factors to malignancies of the large bowel are polyps and ulcerative colitis. Adenocarcinoma of the colon and rectum develops as a polypoid or annular constrictive neoplasm. The annular adenocarcinoma proliferates and grows around the colon and rectum causing a decrease in the size of the lumen. The polypoid adenocarcinoma projects as a cauliflower-like mass into the lumen of the colon and rectum producing obstruction. The colon above the obstruction becomes dilated. Chronic obstruction develops in the advanced stage of carcinoma of the colon.

Metastases from adenocarcinoma of the large intestines commonly occur to the regional lymph nodes and liver. Malignant neoplasms of the abdomen spread by way of the circulation resulting in metastatic liver involvement. Metastases from the large bowel also occur to the lung, adrenal gland and brain.

DISEASES OF THE PERITONEUM

Inflammation. *Acute peritonitis* is an inflammation of all or part of the peritoneum. Bacteria or chemical agents are generally the etiology of acute peritonitis; however, multiple initiating extrinsic and intrinsic factors may be present. Bile and gastric juice are chemicals which are capable of producing peritonitis. The organisms responsible for provoking peritonitis are *Bacillus coli,* non-hemolytic streptococci, diphtheroid bacillus, *Bacillus lactis aerogenes, Bacillus melanogenicum,* pneumococcus and hemolytic streptococcus. There are four possible routes of entry of bacteria into the peritoneum, i.e. by way of the blood stream, vagina and fallopian tube, wall of the gastrointestinal tract, and transdiaphragmatic as a complication of pulmonary diseases.

Grossly, there is generally some type of peritoneal exudate which ranges from a serous to a purulent and fibrinous exudate. Peritonitis produces chills, fever and leukocytosis, stimulation of nerve endings leading to pain, pain resulting in muscle spasm in the abdominal wall and rigidity, the presence of the exudate in the peritoneal cavity which helps to distend the abdomen, inhibited intestinal motility, and nausea and vomiting.

MISCELLANEOUS DISTURBANCES OF THE GASTROINTESTINAL TRACT

Hernia. Hernia is the protusion of an entire viscus or its wall through the enclosing wall. An abdominal hernia can be reduced. A hernia may be internal or external, and acquired or congenital.

Intersussception. Intersussception is an invagination of one loop into another loop of the bowel. In children intersussception is due to the enlargement of a lymph follicle or to local persistence of peristalsis. In adults intersussception occurs secondary to pedunculated neoplasms and thickened bowel walls.

Volvulus. Volvulus is a twisting of the sigmoid colon or small intestines. The mesenteric vessels are compressed resulting in infarction and gangrene. The prognosis and mortality depend upon the length of time that the volvulus has been present.

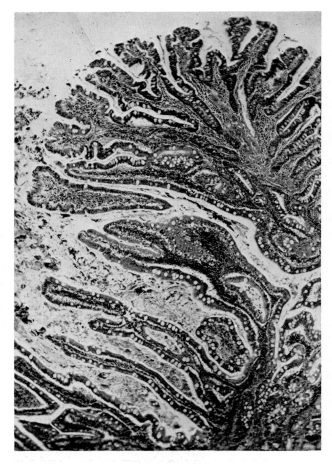

Figure 53. Peutz-Jeghers syndrome. Notice the multiple polyposis of the small bowel. The polyposis is familial and is accompanied by focal melanin pigmentation of the oral mucosa and skin.

Intestinal Polyposis (Peutz-Jeghers Syndrome). Peutz-Jeghers syndrome is an inherited syndrome consisting of multiple fibromas, polyposis of the small bowel, and focal melanin pigmentation of the oral mucosa and lips. The polyposis associated with the Peutz-Jeghers syndrome are benign lesions which only rarely become malignant.

Chapter 15

DISEASES OF THE LIVER AND BILIARY TRACT

The liver functions as a chemical laboratory and performs the following functions: (1) bile production and excretion; (2) metabolism of fats, carbohydrates, vitamins, and mineral metabolism; (3) storage of vitamins A, C and D; (4) chemical detoxification by hepatic cells; (5) reticuloendothelial participation in detoxification by means of phagocytosis by kupffer cells; and (6) hematopoiesis and coagulation by means of storage of vitamin B_{12} and vitamin K.

Bile is produced by the liver and passes into the duodenum. Bile aids in the emulsification of fat along with the action of lipase which prepares the fat for absorption. Vitamins A and K are fat soluble vitamins, therefore, when fat is decreased or absent, vitamins A and K are not absorbed. Bile contains bilirubin, bile salts and cholesterol. The bile salts are formed in the liver. Cholesterol is produced and eliminated by the liver. Bilirubin is derived from the breakdown of hemoglobin.

DEGENERATIVE CHANGES IN THE LIVER

Fatty Change. Fatty change produces a greasy, yellow-colored liver. Microscopically, the liver cord cells contain large, clear vacuoles located in the cytoplasm. The fat vacuole pushes the centrally located nucleus to the periphery of the cell.

Chronic Passive Congestion. During chronic passive congestion, the liver is hyperemic in the area of the central veins. Compression of liver cords occurs with atrophy of hepatic cells. Central lobular necrosis is the result of chronic passive congestion.

Infarction. Infarction is rare but may occur in the liver when complete obstruction is present in the portal vein or hepatic artery located in the portal triad. Complete necrosis does not occur in the liver because of the double circulation to this organ. Partial necrosis occurs when an obstruction is present in either the portal vein or hepatic artery. If an obstruction occurs to the portal vein before it enters the liver, no infarction results because the hepatic artery provides the blood supply. However, if the obstruction develops suddenly, infarction will occur in an organ (liver) with a double blood supply.

Infarction of the liver is, therefore, rare for the following reasons: (1) double blood supply; (2) 65 percent of the blood supply occurs by way of the portal vein; (3) the liver is resistant to relative anoxia; (4) collateral

143

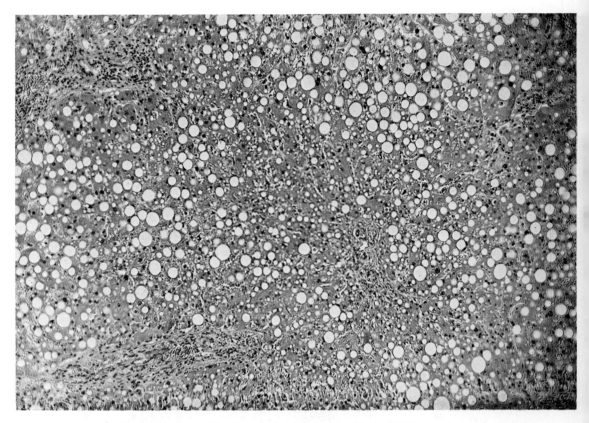

Figure 54. Fatty change of the liver. Notice the accumulation of fat in the hepatic cells where no fat is evident histologically.

vessels pass from the diaphragm to the liver; and (5) the hepatic artery does not arise directly from the aorta. The liver has a limited ability to regenerate parenchymal cells.

Amyloidosis. Amyloidosis of the liver produces stiff margins and overall increase in the size of the organ.

Necrosis. Five types of liver necrosis may be identified, i.e. *central zonal, midzonal, peripheral zonal, focal* and *diffuse necrosis.* Central zonal necrosis of the liver is due to anoxia, chronic passive hyperemia, chemical poisons, and acute viral hepatitis.

The most common necrosis occurs around the central vein. Midzonal necrosis of the liver is due to yellow fever, infectious diseases, burns, and tannic acid. The rare peripheral zonal necrosis is due to eclampsia and phosphorus poisoning. Focal necrosis of the liver is due to typhoid fever and other infectious diseases. Diffuse necrosis of the liver is due to syphilis, Weil's disease, viral hepatitis and acute yellow atrophy.

When a large quantity of poison is consumed, or if liver disease or congestive heart failure is present, acute yellow atrophy of the liver occurs rather than the zonal type of necrosis. Chemicals and drugs which are directly toxic to the liver may provoke a hypersensitivity reaction, i.e. a focal type of liver

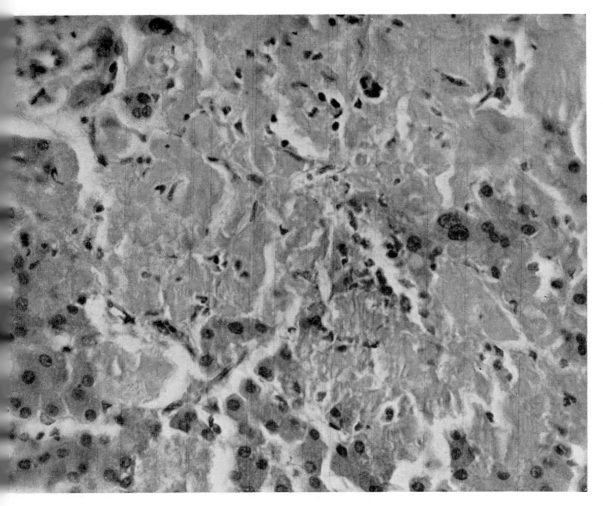

Figure 55. Amyloidosis of the liver. Notice the marked deposition of amyloid in the liver. The amyloid causes pressure atrophy and degeneration of hepatic parenchymal cells.

necrosis. Bacterial toxins accompanied by a generalized septicemia result in focal areas of necrosis in the liver.

Cholangitis is produced when organisms reach the liver through the portal vein resulting in infection of the biliary tract and bile ducts. The infection spreads through the liver producing abscesses in the parenchyma.

INFECTIONS OF THE LIVER

Infectious agents may reach the liver by direct extension in the event of trauma or from an infection in the peritoneal cavity. Rarely do infectious agents reach the liver by way of the portal vein or hepatic artery. Any infection in the spleen and gastrointestinal tract (rarely intestinal infection) may lead to liver damage by means of bacterial or septic emboli. The liver is a fairly resistant organ which contains phagocytic cells of the reticuloendo-thelial system. When infection takes place in the liver, the microorganisms

CIRRHOSIS OF THE LIVER

Cirrhosis of the liver refers to the development of fibrosis, i.e. scarring of the liver. Cirrhosis is a chronic disease process which is progressive and dynamic rather than static. The fibrosis is diffuse and may involve every lobule of the liver by connective tissue which causes disruption of the normal architecture of the liver. There are three forms of cirrhosis based on morphologic characteristics, i.e. portal (Laennac's) cirrhosis, postnecrotic cirrhosis, and biliary cirrhosis. The most common portal atrophy (Laennac's cirrhosis) is related to protein, sulfur containing amino acid, choline, cystine, and methionine nutritional deficiencies. A choline deficient diet and a methionine deficient diet result in a fatty liver and cirrhosis.

Portal Cirrhosis (Laennec's Cirrhosis). Portal cirrhosis occurs in approximately 2 to 3 percent of the population of the United States. The age distribution in the United States is from forty to sixty years. Portal cirrhosis is more common in males than in females. Portal cirrhosis shows a higher incidence in the Negro than in the Caucasian. The etiology of portal cirrhosis is obscure. Fifty percent of patients with portal cirrhosis give a history of alcoholism. However, many alcoholics never have portal cirrhosis. Protein, carbohydrate and vitamin deficiencies (malnutrition), and infectious diseases are etiologic factors.

During portal cirrhosis the liver is generally smaller than normal and is firm, nodular and yellow in color. The cut section of the liver reveals fine nodules with a yellow color to both the cut and capsular surfaces. The liver has a tough consistency and cuts with increased resistance.

The clinical features of portal cirrhosis include the following: dyspepsia, anorexia, lower abdominal pain, constipation, tenderness in right hypergastric region (upper gastric region), amenorrhea, sterility in males, gynecomastia, and terminal edema and jaundice. The most important clinical feature of portal cirrhosis is ascites. The liver is palpable in 80 percent and the spleen is palpable in 50 percent of patients with portal cirrhosis.

Diffuse fibrosis is present; however, it is more conspicuous in the portal areas which become attached to one another. Regenerative activity is evident and binucleated cells are present with darkly stained nuclei. Ten to fifteen times the normal number of small bile ducts are present in the portal areas during portal cirrhosis. New bile ducts proliferate in all forms of cirrhosis.

Bile stasis may be present in portal cirrhosis. Bile plugs occur in canaliculi, bilirubin is located in liver cells, and there is destruction of blood and bile circulation. Jaundice occurs in approximately 10 to 20 percent of individuals with portal cirrhosis.

Ascites develops early in portal cirrhosis. Portal hypertension occurs due to the anastomosis between the portal vein and hepatic artery with an increase in pressure. The damaged liver fails in its function of detoxification.

Hyperestrogen, gynecomastia and increased intra-abdominal pressure accompany the failure of detoxification and an increase in hormones.

Biliary Cirrhosis. Biliary cirrhosis is not as common as portal cirrhosis. Biliary cirrhosis is due to obstruction of the bile duct system and alterations in the biliary system. The biliary obstruction may be intrahepatic or result from an obstruction outside of the liver (posthepatic biliary cirrhosis).

Posthepatic biliary cirrhosis is due to a pancreatic carcinoma, gallstone or stricture. In posthepatic biliary cirrhosis the liver is enlarged terminally. In postnecrotic biliary cirrhosis the obstruction causes stasis in the large bile ducts (polystasis). Inflammation occurs secondarily to the polystasis.

Hypertrophic biliary cirrhosis is due to a primary cholangitis of the small branches of bile ducts. The portal areas contain a proliferation of connective tissue, a prominent inflammatory exudate, and proliferation of bile capillaries. Hepatic cell atrophy is a result of the pressure exerted by the fibrosis, interference with the circulation, and anoxia. The normal architecture of the liver is subsequently replaced by pseudolobular formation due to the periportal cirrhosis.

Differentiation of intrahepatic from the extrahepatic type of biliary cirrhosis is possible since the large bile ducts contain bile thrombi in the extrahepatic type. When the etiology of the biliary cirrhosis is intrahepatic in origin, bile thrombi are present in the small bile ducts.

When biliary cirrhosis is due to hyperlipemia and hypercholesterolemia, yellow xanthomas develop on the lower extremities and eyelids.

Postnecrotic Cirrhosis. Postnecrotic cirrhosis follows necrosis of hepatic

TABLE XXI
CLINICAL SIGNS AND LABORATORY FINDINGS IN BILIARY AND PORTAL CIRRHOSIS

Biliary Cirrhosis
  Clinical Signs
    Occurs at any age
    Occurs predominantly in females
    Not associated with alcoholism
    Malnutrition is rare
    Jaundice present (mild to marked)
    Xanthomas present
    None or late hyperestrogen in urine and gynecomastia present
    Ascites absent or occurs late
    Intrahepatic obstruction
    Inspissated bile in canaliculi
    Monolobular cirrhosis (primary)
    Secondary cirrhosis due to carcinoma of the head of pancreas, stone in bile duct or
    Benign stricture of bile duct

  Laboratory Findings
    Marked anemia
    High serum alkaline phosphatase
    High serum cholesterol
    Increased serum phospholipids
    Normal or increased serum proteins
    Decreased serum albumen
    Markedly increased gamma globulin

Portal Cirrhosis
  Clinical Signs
    Occurs between 40 and 60 years of age
    Occurs predominantly in males
    50 percent of individuals are alcoholic
    Malnutrition is present
    Jaundice occurs late (not marked)
    Xanthomas are absent
    Hyperestrogen in urine and gynecomastia present
    Ascites occurs early
    Metaplasia of prostate gland
    Testicular atrophy
    Enlarge spleen
    Esophageal, epigastric and mesenteric varicosities, hemorrhoids

  Laboratory Findings
    Slight anemia (occurs late)
    Normal alkaline phosphatase
    Normal cholesterol (decreased esters)
    Normal or decreased phospholipids
    Decreased serum proteins
    Early decreased serum albumen
    Increased gamma globulin

cells. Infectious agents, toxins, poisons and malnutrition may lead to massive necrosis. Alcoholism plus portal cirrhosis predispose the liver to development of large areas of necrosis. Grossly, the liver is reduced in size. Large irregular nodules are present which represent regenerated liver cells. Irregular broad areas or bands of fibrosis extend into the liver lobule due to the postnecrotic changes.

Cardiac Cirrhosis. Cardiac cirrhosis is associated with pericarditis and rheumatic heart disease. Central lobular dilatation and chronic passive congestion leads to central lobular necrosis. The reticulum collapses and periportal fibrosis results. A fine regular nodularity occurs in cardiac cirrhosis. Less bile duct proliferation takes place and the fibrosis is not marked in cardiac cirrhosis compared to portal cirrhosis.

Cirrhosis with Hemochromatosis. Cirrhosis of the liver accompanied by hemochromatosis is a metabolic disorder resulting in increased absorption of iron and deposition of iron in the liver, pancreas, lymph nodes, skin and other organs. Severe fibrosis occurs in the pancreas which is responsible for producing diabetes mellitus. The skin is pigmented and the alteration is termed *bronzed diabetes*. The liver is enlarged and colored brown due to the tremendous deposition of iron pigment, hemosiderin and hemofuscin. Fibrosis occurs predominantly in the portal region and is multilobular in distribution.

Parasitic Cirrhosis. Parasitic cirrhosis is due to hepatic infection by the

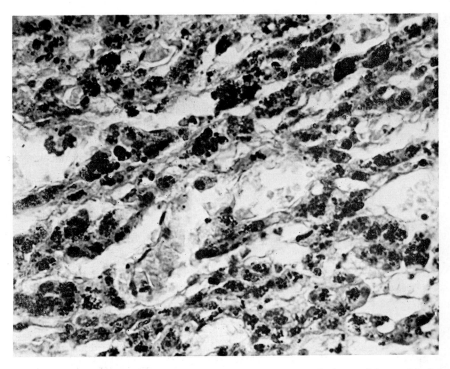

Figure 56. Hemochromatosis of the liver. Notice the accumulations of hemosiderin predominantly located in the hepatic cells at the periphery of hepatic lobules.

liver fluke (*Clonorchis sinensis*) or schistosomiasis. The parasites obstruct the blood stream producing portal cirrhosis and/or the bile ducts producing biliary cirrhosis. Malarial parasites produce portal cirrhosis.

Wilson's Disease. Wilson's disease is a chronic disease due to hepatolenticular degeneration. Three basic findings are present in Wilson's disease, i.e. portal cirrhosis, degeneration of basal ganglion in the brain, and green pigmentation at the outer edge of the cornea.

NEOPLASMS OF THE LIVER

Benign neoplasms of the liver are uncommon. The most important benign neoplasms of the liver are the hemangioma and the adenoma. The adenoma is a cholangioma derived from bile ducts.

Primary carcinoma may occur in the liver. The primary carcinoma of the liver occurs in individuals from fifty to sixty years of age and is more common in males than females. Cirrhosis of the liver is an etiologic factor in primary carcinoma of the liver. The primary carcinoma of the liver occurs in two histologic types, i.e. the hepatocarcinoma and cholangiocarcinoma. The hepatocarcinoma causes an enlarged liver which may be multinodular or diffusely infiltrated with neoplastic cells. The hepatocarcinoma is the most frequent carcinoma of the liver and consists of neoplastic cells situated in columns similar to hepatic cords and abnormal lobule formation. The clinical features of primary carcinoma of the liver are pain, dyspepsia, weight loss, enlarged liver, enlarged pigmented spleen, and jaundice (80% of patients).

DISEASES OF THE BILIARY TRACT

Inflammation, neoplasia and lithiasis are the principal pathologic processes which involve the biliary tract. The hepatic duct passes downward from the liver to join the cystic duct in forming the common bile duct (common hepatic duct). The common bile duct joins the pancreatic duct forming the ampulla of Vater just proximal to their site of entrance into the duodenum. Bile is secreted by the liver and concentrated in the gall bladder. Bile contains bile salts, bile pigments (bilirubin and biliverdin), alkali carbonates, cholesterol, mucin and water. If equilibrium of bile constituents is not maintained, a deposition of elements takes place providing a nidus for the formation of stones.

Inflammation of the Gall Bladder. Bacteria may enter the gall bladder by way of the blood stream or biliary system. Microorganisms grow in the biliary system if there is stasis of bile or if an obstruction is present. *Acute cholecystitis* may occur due to bacterial infection with streptococci, staphylococci, *Eschericia coli* and typhi. Acute cholecystitis may occur as a nonbacterial inflammation due to increased retention of bile salts. The infection starts in the mucosa and extends into the wall of the gall bladder.

Chronic Cholecystitis. Chronic cholecystitis may occur as chronic inflammation from the start or the acute disease may become chronic. A thick fibrosed gall bladder with adhesions and areas of inflammation and necrosis occur in chronic cholecystitis. Cholecystitis is responsible for the formation of gallstones.

Cholesterolosis is a strawberry gall bladder containing seed-like spots on the surface. The yellow areas are due to masses of cholesterol esters which are deposited in the mucosal lining and in deeper areas of the wall of the gall bladder.

Empyema of Gall Bladder. Empyema is the accumulation of pus in the gall bladder due to a severe infection and obstruction. The lumen is distended, mucosal folds are obliterated, and an exudate covers the mucosa.

Hydrops of the Gall Bladder. When obstruction occurs to the passage of bile from the gall bladder, in the absence of infection, the gall bladder becomes distended with mucin. The mucin plugs the ducts and the gall bladder becomes distended with white bile (mucin), i.e. hydrops of the gall bladder.

Cholelithiasis. Cholelithiasis is the formation and presence of gallstones in the gall bladder and bile passages including the bile ducts of the liver. *Pure cholesterol gallstones* develop as solitary stones termed *metabolic stones*. *Pure calcium bilirubinate gallstones* develop in hemolytic jaundice as multiple stones due to increased hemolysis. Calcium bilirubinate stones are black, friable, multiple small stones. Ten percent of patients with hemolytic jaundice develop calcium bilirubinate stones. *Pure calcium carbonate gallstones* form rare solitary gray amorphous stones. *Mixed cholelithiasis* form as multiple faceted stones. Ten percent of all cholelithiases are pure stones and 90 percent are mixed faceted multiple stones associated with infection.

The etiologic factors in the formation of cholelithiasis include the following: infection, stasis of bile, high serum cholesterol, and high bile cholesterol. The most common complications of cholelithiasis include obstruction, perforation of the ileum or colon, ulceration, and formation of a fistula.

Neoplasms of the Gall Bladder. *Papillomas* occur in the neck of the gall bladder. *Adenomas* and *adenomyomas* occur in the fundus of the gall bladder. Malignant neoplasms of the gall bladder are associated with long standing cholelithiasis and are more common in females than in males. Carcinoma occurs in the neck or fundus of the gall bladder. The neoplastic cells infiltrate the wall of the gall bladder and are responsible for ulceration of areas of the mucosa.

The *adenocarcinoma* is the predominant carcinoma of the gall bladder. Metastasis takes place to the liver and to the area surrounding the gall bladder. Obstructive jaundice and biliary cirrhosis occur following metastases. *Squamous cell carcinoma* of the gall bladder is rare. It is due to metaplasia of the epithelium due to long standing irritation from cholelithiasis.

Chapter 16

DISEASES OF THE LYMPH NODES AND SPLEEN

DISEASES OF THE LYMPH NODES

Inflammatory Diseases of the Lymph Nodes. Lymph nodes contain reticuloendothelial cells which act as a filtering system to remove irritants which pass to the lymph node by way of the lymphatics. *Acute lymphadenitis* is the most common alteration of lymph nodes.

Lymphadenitis may develop in those lymph nodes draining any region of acute inflammation. The lymph nodes become enlarged and tender or painful. The enlargement of lymph nodes during acute lymphadenitis is due to hyperplasia of the cellular elements and infiltration of acute inflammatory cells. Diphtheria, pharyngitis, measles, scarlet fever, gastroenteritis, vaginitis, pyogenic infection and abscess, cellulitis, and mononucleosis are representative of the wide range of pathologic processes associated with localized and generalized acute lymphadenitis.

The enlarged lymph nodes due to acute lymphadenitis may persist for several weeks and in children the enlargement is commonly accompanied by fever, fluctuations, convulsions and meningitis.

Chronic lymphadenitis occurs in lymph nodes draining areas of low-grade inflammation. The nodes show proliferation of mononuclear cells. The lymph nodes do not reach a large size during chronic lymphadenitis.

Chronic granulomatous lymphadenitis is due to tuberculosis, sarcoidosis, cat-scratch disease, lymphopathia venereum, brucellosis and tularemia. The lymph nodes show areas of necrosis and proliferation of epithelioid histiocytic cells and hyperplasia of reticulum cells.

Infectious mononucleosis is a contagious disease affecting the cervical lymph nodes. During infectious mononucleosis immature white blood cells, probably lymphoblasts, are present in the circulating blood.

Neoplasms of Lymph Nodes. The *malignant lymphomas* comprise neoplastic pathologic processes involving the lymph nodes of the body. The *giant follicle lymphosarcoma* is a malignant lymphoma of lymph nodes and lymphoid tissues. The neoplasm produces a prominent follicular pattern. The large follicles are closely packed together and a condensation of reticulum fibers is present at the periphery of follicles. The enlarged follicles are located in the peripheral area as well as in the central zone of the lymph nodes. In the advanced stage of this lymphoma the follicular pattern disappears.

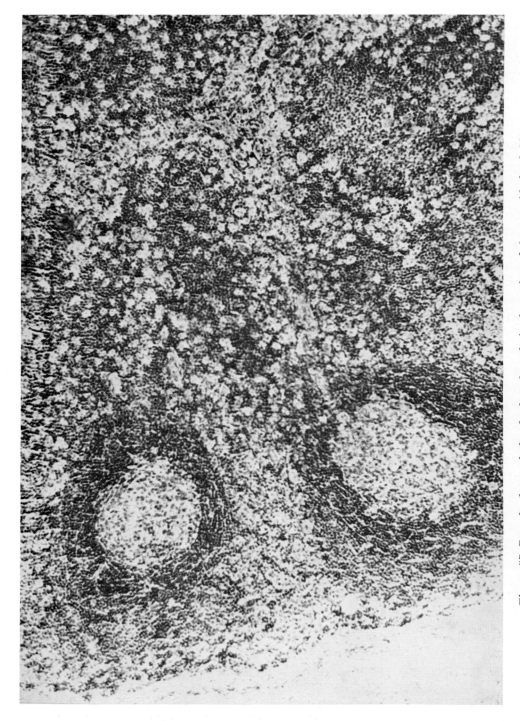

Figure 57. Reactive hyperplasia of a lymph node in the region of the parotid gland. Notice the sharply-outlined reactive follicles. Lymphocytes are present at the margin of the reactive follicles. The centers of the follicles are composed of uniform reticulum cells.

Lymphosarcoma is a malignant lymphoma of the lymph nodes which arises from lymphoid tissue at a mean age of forty-five years. Lymphadenopathy occurs early in this lymphoma with the cervical lymph nodes most commonly involved. Extension to other lymph nodes occurs in the early stage of this neoplasm. Metastasis takes place later by way of the blood stream to affect various organs throughout the body. The lymphosarcoma arises from the undifferentiated mesenchymal cell of the lymph node. Lymphosarcoma has been classified into the following: lymphocytic variety composed of well differentiated small lymphocytes, lymphoblastic variety composed of undifferentiated large lymphocytes, mixed variety composed of lymphocytes and reticulum cells, and reticulum cell variety (reticulum cell sarcoma).

Reticulum cell sarcoma is a malignant lymphoma of lymph nodes of obscure etiology. The sarcoma may be localized or generalized and the affected individual loses weight, and develops fever and anemia. The reticulum cell sarcoma is commonly present in the visceral lymph nodes causing displacement of the kidney, stomach and intestines. The affected lymph nodes become matted together into one syncytium.

The lymphosarcoma destroys the normal architecture of the lymph node due to proliferation of neoplastic cells. Lymphoblasts proliferate and destroy the sinuses of the affected lymph nodes. The neoplastic cells are similar in morphology, penetrate the capsule of the node and invade the adjacent structures.

Lymphatic leukemia is a form of malignant lymphoma which involves the lymph nodes. Lymphatic leukemia is accompanied by fever, anemia, and lymph node enlargement. Lymphatic leukemia has a similar morphologic appearance to the lymphosarcoma. The architecture of the lymph nodes is destroyed by small lymphocytes and some large and young neoplastic cells.

Hodgkin's disease is a form of malignant lymphoma involving the lymph nodes or lymphoid tissue in the spleen, gastrointestinal tract, and bone marrow. The etiology of Hodgkin's disease is obscure; however, it has been considered a viral infection, a neoplasm of lymphoid tissue, and a chronic granuloma. Hodgkin's disease is two to three times more common in males than females. It occurs more commonly in individuals between twenty and forty years of age but may occur at any age. Hodgkin's disease is twice as common in young adults as the lymphosarcoma. However, Hodgkin's disease has the same frequency in children as the lymphosarcoma. Hodgkin's disease begins as an enlargement of the cervical lymph nodes in the neck. The enlarged cervical nodes are initially discrete. However, during the late stages of the disease the individual nodes become fused togther. Splenomegaly, hepatomegaly, and anemia are present. In early Hodgkin's disease the lymph nodes are affected by a lymphoblastic hyperplasia. In late Hodgkin's disease a reticulum cell hyperplasia with eosinophils and giant cells is the dominant histopathologic feature. In still a later stage of Hodgkin's disease there is a replacement of the cellular structure of lymph nodes by

TABLE XXII

COMPARISON OF FEATURES OF THE MALIGNANT LYMPHOMAS

Giant Follicular Lymphoma (Lymphoblastoma)

Produces localized lesion
Lymph nodes enlarged
Spleen enlarged late in 30 percent of cases
No bone involvement
Formation of giant follicles in lymph node
Increase in the number of follicles or germinal centers
Hyperplastic germinal cells with mitosis
Coalescence of adjacent follicles
Tendency for follicles to separate from surrounding tissue (artifact)
In late stage follicular structure of nodes is lost
May be cured by surgery
Pancytopenia (rare) due to terminal hypersplenism

Reticulum Cell Sarcoma

Occasionally isolate lesion
More common in lymph nodes compared to lymphosarcoma
Large neoplastic reticulum cells have infolded large nucleus and abundant cytoplasm
Sarcoma infiltrates veins
There may or may not be an increase in reticulum in lymph nodes
Reticulum fibers encircle groups of reticulum cells with cytoplasmic processes suggesting reticulum origin
Polymorphous giant cells of a bizarre type

Hodgkin's Disease

A fatal malignant lymphoma
Status considered neoplastic or inflammatory disease
Two or three times more common in males than females
Twice as common in adults as lymphosarcoma
Same incidence in children as lymphosarcoma
Deep and superficial cervical lymph nodes most commonly enlarged
Mediastinal, mesenteric and retroperitoneal lymph nodes also enlarged (any lymph node may be involved)
Splenomegaly accompanies 50 to 75 percent of instances of Hodgkin's disease
Hepatomegaly—gray areas present in portal tracts
Anemia
Megakaryocytes in blood
Fever
Pruritus (itching)
Pigmentation
Groups of nodes are continuous with one another
There is invasion of tissue surrounding nodes
Nodes are grossly fish-flesh and homogeneous
Hodgkin's tissue, termed suet areas, occurs in spleen
There is a multiplicity of cell types in Hodgkin's tissue of lymph nodes
Pleomorphism of reticulum cells suggests inflammation
Reed-Sternberg cells (Multinucleated giant reticulum cells)

Proliferation of pale large reticuloendothelial cells (epithelioid cells)
Eosinophilic leukocytes most conspicuous in nodes
Increase in reticulum in nodes
Fibrosis in late stage of Hodgkin's disease
Plasma cells, neutrophiles, fibroblasts, and tissue necrosis present in lymph nodes
Bone marrow is hyperplastic, contains an accumulation of large mononuclear cells which arise from reticulum cells, multinucleated giant cells, eosinophiles, necrosis and progressive fibrosis in late stage of disease
Bone marrow involved in 20 percent of cases of Hodgkin's disease

Lymphosarcoma

Lymph nodes enlarged
Spleen enlarged in 50 percent of cases
Groups of lymph nodes are continuous with one another
Lymphocytosis
Tendency for lymphoblastic and lymphocytic cells to rupture through capsule and invade surrounding tissue
Diffuse proliferation of cells, normal structures of lymph node are obscure
Necrosis minimal
Normal lymphocytes replaced by large hyperchromatic cells with small quantity of cytoplasm and prominent nucleoli
Mitosis may or may not be common
There is uniformity of cell type
No increase in reticulum
Neoplastic cells strikingly uniform in appearance
Undifferentiated type termed lymphoblastic lymphosarcoma
Differentiated type termed lymphocytic lymphocarcoma
Bone involved in 20 percent of cases
Blood is rarely involved; however, leukemia may occur rarely in the terminal stage

Lymphatic Leukemia

Generalized enlargement of lymph nodes
Deep and superficial lymph nodes enlarged in 90% of cases
Lymph nodes overrun with lymphocytes
Patients may live an extended period of time
In myelogenous leukemia lymph node involvement is not as common as in lymphatic leukemia
White blood cell count 50,000 to 200,000
Lymphocytosis 85 percent with small-size prolymphocytes dominant
Decreased platelets
Focal or nodular accumulation of lymphocytes may occur in bone marrow
Obliteration of normal architecture of lymph nodes, loss of germinal centers and lymph sinuses, loss of distinction between cortex and medulla of node
Mitosis may be present
Capsule of node is infiltrated with lymphocytic cells and neoplastic cells invade surrounding tissue

Table XXII (*Continued*)

Phagocytes are present in involved lymph nodes

In chronic lymphatic leukemia the neoplastic cells approach small lymphocytes; however, larger and younger cells are present

Bone tissue is not generally involved except in 10% of cases where bone destruction takes place due to infiltration of lymphocytes in bone marrow

Spleen involved in 80 to 85 percent of instances of lymphatic leukemia

Hodgkin's Sarcoma

Histopathology—uniform large neoplastic cells with abundant cytoplasm and large prominent nucleus, mitosis, and no formation of reticulum

fibrous connective tissue producing a hard and contracted lymph node. The architecture of the affected lymph node is obliterated in all instances of Hodgkin's disease. The lymphoblastic proliferation of early Hodgkin's disease may be confused with the lymphosarcoma. The pleomorphism of reticulum cells suggests that Hodgkin's disease may be an infective granuloma. Large pale reticuloendothelial cells (epithelioid cells), Reed-Sternberg multinucleated giant cells, and fibrosis in the late stage constitute the histologic features of Hodgkin's disease (Hodgkin's granuloma).

Hodgkin's disease has been classified into the following types on the basis of histopathology, i.e. Hodgkin's paragranuloma, Hodgkin's granuloma, and Hodgkin's sarcoma. Hodgkin's paragranuloma is a benign disease of the cervical lymph nodes producing cervical lymphadenopathy as the main symptom. Hodgkin's paragranuloma may undergo transformation into Hodgkin's granuloma which is probably the commonest variety of Hodgkin's disease. Hodgkin's granuloma is synonymous with Hodgkin's disease. Hodgkin's sarcoma is the most anaplastic variety of the disease. This neoplasm runs a highly malignant course and has the same incidence in males and females between fifty and seventy years of age. Pleomorphic lymphocytic and reticulum cells, mitoses, fibrosis, and the presence of Reed-Sternberg cells are the principal histopathologic findings.

Metastatic Neoplasms to the Lymph Nodes. The metastatic neoplasms to the lymph nodes are much more common than the primary lymphomas. The majority of metastatic neoplasms to lymph nodes are epithelial in origin. The metastatic cells in the lymph nodes may be either the same degree of differentiation or less differentiated than the cells of the primary neoplasm.

DISEASES OF THE SPLEEN

The spleen is a vascular organ which represents the largest single collection of lymphoid and reticuloendothelial tissues in the body. The spleen has the function of detaining and altering the blood as it passes through the organ. The spleen is a filter for bacteria and hemolyzed red blood cells. The spleen is capable of production of blood cells (extramedullary hematopoesis).

Anomalies of the Spleen. An *accessory spleen* is an anomaly of principal interest to surgeons since it may be overlooked during splenectomy in the treatment of primary splenic disease.

Retrograde Changes in the Spleen. *Amyloidosis* is a degenerative irreversible change in the spleen characterized by deposition of amyloid either locally or diffusely causing splenomegaly. Focal necrosis, atrophy and pigmentation may occur in the spleen. *Rupture* of the spleen may occur spontaneously or result from trauma. Splenic rupture is characterized by a possible history of splenomegaly or injury followed by a sudden onset of abdominal pain, non-shifting paravertebral dullness, increasing anemia, decrease in hematocrit, and leukocytosis. A ruptured spleen may be associated with typhoid fever, malaria and infectious mononucleosis.

Circulatory Disturbances in the Spleen. Chronic *passive hyperemia* produces a congested and enlarged spleen as a result of mitral valve disease or in following portal obstruction. *Infarction* of the spleen is caused by embolic occlusion of a branch of the splenic artery. Infarction of the spleen is usually associated with subacute bacterial endocarditis and leukemia.

Banti's syndrome (splenic anemia) includes enlargement of the spleen, nonhemolytic anemia, leukopenia, and there may or may not be portal cirrhosis. The enlarged spleen is congested and fibrotic. Hemorrhages develop and precede the fibrosis. Dilated splenic sinusoids are present with thick, collagenous walls. The original lesion in Banti's syndrome may be cirrhosis of the liver.

Felty's syndrome is a symptom complex consisting of enlargement of the spleen in adults, chronic arthritis with leukopenia, and lymphadenopathy.

Hemolytic jaundice is an inherited and congenital disease transmitted as a Mendelian dominant characteristic. Hemolytic jaundice is characterized by an enlarged spleen, jaundice, fever, and spheroid-shaped erythrocytes with increased fragility (spherocytic anemia). The splenic enlargement is the result of hypertrophy of phagocytic cells and the accumulation of blood in the splenic pulp.

Pernicious anemia is accompanied by an enlarged spleen with hemosiderin pigment deposited in the splenic pulp. *Polycythemia vera* is accompanied by vascular thrombosis and excessive red blood cells in the enlarged spleen. The thrombosis may cause splenic infarcts producing abdominal pain.

Inflammation of the Spleen. *Acute splenitis (acute splenic tumor)* is characterized by an enlarged and tender spleen which accompanies bacteremias or septicemias. The softest spleen occurs during septicemia and pyemia. The enlarged spleen results from a proliferation of mononuclear cells, blood and hyperplastic follicles.

Myeloid metaplasia of the spleen is characterized clinically by anemia, pallor, slight icterus, splenomegaly, hepatomegaly and bone pain. The affected individual has a history of polycythemia vera or diseases of bone tissue. The bone marrow is acellular and fibrotic. The splenomegaly may be due to the development of active hematopoietic tissue in the spleen.

Neoplasms of the Spleen. *Hodgkin's disease* causes an enlarged spleen since it represents a disease of the reticuloendothelial system. All forms of *leukemia* produce splenomegaly. The lymphoid reticuloendothelial cells proliferate and the sinuses of the spleen are filled with leukemic cells. *Lymphosarcoma* results in infiltration of the splenic parenchyma with neoplastic lymphoid cells and prolymphocytes.

Lipidosis of the Reticuloendothelial System. The lipidosis are rare lipid storage diseases and are characterized by an accumulation of lipids in varying quantities in reticuloendothelial cells, i.e. Gaucher's disease and Niemann-Pick disease. A non-lipid reticuloendotheliosis or osseous xanthomatosis termed *Hand-Schüller-Christian syndrome* also affects the spleen.

Gaucher's disease is a chronic familial cerebroside lipoidosis in which kerasin accumulates abnormally in the reticulum cells of the spleen, lymph nodes, liver and bone marrow. The disease is initiated during childhood and continues for many years into adulthood. Massive enlargement of the spleen occurs. The lymph nodes are only moderately enlarged. The spleen contains collections of large mononuclear cells filled with kerasin. The large pale mononuclear cells are termed *Gaucher cells*. The latter cells accumulate and cause the excessive enlargement of the spleen.

Niemann-Pick Disease. Niemann-Pick disease is a lipidosis due to the abnormal accumulation of sphingomyelin in reticuloendothelial cells and histiocytic cells of tissues and organs. The disease occurs in young infants and is fatal by two years of age. Lipid-filled cells are present in the spleen, lymph nodes, liver and bone marrow. However, the sphingomyelin containing cells may be present in the lung, adrenal, thyroid, brain, pancreas and

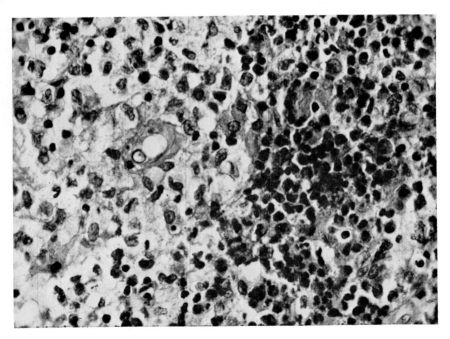

Figure 58. Reticuloendotheliosis (histiocytosis X). Notice the diffuse hyperplasia of elements of the reticuloendothelial system with obliteration of the normal architecture of the tissue. There is a proliferation of large mononuclear histiocytes. Eosinophilic leukocytes are present adjacent to the large histiocytes.

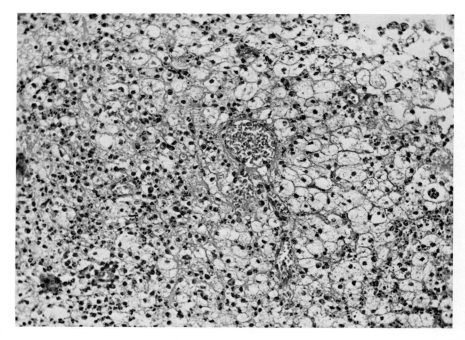

Figure 59. Hand-Schüller-Christian's disease of bone. Notice the localized accumulations of large round mononuclear phagocytic cells containing cholesterol.

glomeruli of the kidney. Deposition of sphingomyelin in the ganglion cells of the brain may result in idiocy.

Hand-Schüller-Christian Syndrome is basically an osseous xanthomatosis in children and adults. The symptom complex includes defects of membranous bones, diabetes insipidus, and exophthalmos. Defects are common in the skeleton, particularly in the skull. The latter defects consist of collections of xanthoma cells which contain cholesterol. The cholesterol accumulates in phagocytic cells of the reticuloendothelial system.

Chapter 17

DISEASES OF THE HEMATOPOIETIC SYSTEM: BLOOD AND BONE MARROW

INTRODUCTION TO DISEASES OF THE BLOOD AND BONE MARROW

Blood formation starts in the liver after the second month of intrauterine life and continues for a period following birth. The spleen participates in blood formation after the second month of intrauterine life and continues until the seventh month of fetal life. Eventually the marrow takes over the function of hematopoiesis. All of the bone marrow throughout the body is red or hematopoietic bone marrow until puberty. At puberty there is a regression of active bone marrow. Hematopoietic bone is located in the ribs, vertebrate, distal portion of the femur, humerus, sternum, and innominate bones. All blood cells are formed in the bone marrow. The entire circulating red blood cells and their precursors originate in the bone marrow. Oxygen is carried by the hemoglobin. Approximately 15 different chemical types of hemoglobin have been described.

ALTERATIONS IN RED BLOOD CELLS

Loss of hemoglobin and decrease in the number of red blood cells results in anemia. The general morphology of the organs of the body during anemia depends upon the severity and duration of the disease.

Anemias Due to Blood Loss. Anemias may be due to loss of blood from the body. Chronic hemorrhage leads to chronic anemia. In chronic anemia the nails are brittle and spoon shaped. Cardiac cells, epithelial cells of renal tubules, hepatic cells, and ganglion cells of the central nervous system show fatty degeneration.

Hemolytic anemias are due to extrinsic factors, i.e. bacterial toxins, antigens, or hematologic injury to red blood cells. Intrinsic factors also produce hemolytic anemias due to anoxia. When rapid hemolysis occurs the result is acute tubular necrosis, hemosiderosis and hyperplastic normoblastic bone marrow.

Spherocytic anemia (congenital hemolytic anemia) is a congenital, familial, Mendelian dominant disease which becomes clinically evident early in life. There is an inherent defect in the red blood cells which affects individuals of any race and in both sexes. The disease is characterized by prolonged or recurrent attacks of jaundice accompanied by varying degrees of anemia and splenomegaly. The red blood cells are biconvex discs (sphero-cytes) and show excessive fragility and decreased resistance.

The spleen is enlarged, congested, and contains enlarged sinusoids. Foci of extramedullary hematopoiesis develop in the liver and excessive hemo-siderin pigment is present in the bone marrow and parenchymal organs. Proliferative changes occur in the outer plate of the skull producing the tower skull. The clinical finding of spherocytic anemia include mild jaun-dice, high incidence of gall stones, chronic leg ulcers, and hemorrhage that may occur into the intestines.

Sickle cell anemia is a congenital hemolytic anemia transmitted as a Men-delian dominant hereditary characteristic. Sickle cell anemia is present in approximately 7 to 10 percent of Negroes in the United States. The disease occurs in young adults of either sex. The sickle cell trait produces sickled red blood cells, i.e. the formation of bizarre shaped cells when exposed to low oxygen tension. The sickling of red blood cells is due to the presence of hemoglobin S in individuals with sickle cell anemia. Hemoglobin S is less soluble and crystallizes as compared to normal hemoglobin. In the individ-uals with sickle cell anemia there is less oxygen, more sickling in the venous blood, and the hemoglobin is all hemoglobin S. In the latter individuals the fetal hemoglobin is replaced by hemoglobin S instead of by normal adult hemoglobin A. During a hemolytic crisis the patient will have some fetal hemoglobin, jaundice, leukocytosis, and decreased platelets. The spleen is congested and enlarged. There are recurrent attacks of weakness, fatigue and anemia. Pain occurs in the gastrointestinal tract and nausea and vomiting are present.

Cooley's Mediterranean anemia or thalassemia is a form of erythroblastic anemia. The disease is congenital and familial and occurs among children of the Mediterranean races. The disease is due to the persistence of fetal hemoglobin. The disease follows a severe course and death occurs in child-hood. The clinical features are thickening of the skull and long bones, Mon-goloid facies, enlarged spleen, pallor, and enlarged abdomen due to hep-atomegaly and splenomegaly. There is reduced destruction of blood and less hemosiderosis; however, hemosiderin may be found in the parenchymal organs. Hyperplasia of the bone marrow is present in the porous long bones with thickened cortex.

Erythroblastosis fetalis or hemolytic disease of the newborn is a congenital disease of the newborn in which an excessive quantity of immature red blood cells are present in the peripheral blood. Excessive hemolysis and destruc-tion of red blood cells occur in the peripheral blood. Extramedullary he-matopoiesis is present in the spleen and liver. Red blood cells are present in various tissues of the body. The acute disease of the newborn is characterized by hydrops fetalis, i.e. edema and ascites, icterus gravis neonatorum (intense jaundice), and kernicterus (bile pigmentation of basal ganglia of the brain which accompanies erythroblastic anemia of the newborn).

The Rh factor is important in erythroblastosis fetalis. The child born from an Rh-negative mother and Rh-positive father has a good chance of in-heriting the Rh factor. When the Rh factor is inherited the fetus produces anti-Rh agglutinins in the maternal blood stream. The anti-Rh agglutinins pass through the placenta causing destruction of the red blood cells of the fetus.

Hemoglobinuria is caused by syphilis and exposure to cold. Hemoglobi-nuria is the result of hemolysis of red blood cells intravenously. Moderate splenomegaly and heptomegaly are present and the urine has a clear, port wine color and contains hemolyzed red blood cells. The intravascular release of hemoglobin produces methemoglobin which colors the plasma pink.

Anemias Due to Decreased Red Blood Cell Production. *Hypochromic anemias* result from a deficiency of iron caused by acute or chronic hemor-rhage, chronic infections, parasitic infections, pregnancy, neoplasms, diseases of the gastrointestinal tract, and lead poisoning. When acute hemorrhage occurs in a patient with hypochromic anemia the findings include leuko-cytosis, increased reticulocyte count, and hyperplasia of the normoblasts of bone marrow. The red blood cells are smaller than normal and the hemo-globin concentration is less than 30 percent of normal. The parenchymal or-gans show degenerative changes.

Idiopathic hypochromic anemia occurs in Caucasians; generally females between forty and fifty years of age. The disease has an occasional familial incidence. The findings include normal to slightly reduced red blood cell count, markedly decreased hemoglobin, decreased color index, decreased hematocrit, microcytosis, normal leukocytes, achlorhydria, atrophy of mu-cous membrane and dysphagia. The anemia is progressive with no spontane-ous remissions. Administration of iron is the recommended therapy.

Pernicious anemia is due to a deficiency of the extrinsic factor, i.e. vita-min B_{12} and of the intrinsic factor (unknown substance) produced by cells of the stomach. The gastric deficiency produces gastric achlorhydria and variable gastrointestinal and neurological disturbances. The intrinsic factor is necessary for absorption of vitamin B_{12} from the small intestines.

Pernicious anemia affects both sexes but is more common in males. It occurs in individuals from forty to sixty years of age. Pernicious anemia is chiefly a disease of the Caucasian race (Nordic types). The disease is in-sidious and progresses slowly. The anemia has remissions and exacerbations. The clinical triad of pernicious anemia is weakness, sore tongue, and numb-ness or tingling. The pernicious anemia patient has a lemon yellow pallor, no free hydrochloric acid in the stomach, and gastrointestinal and central nervous system symptoms. The blood picture in pernicious anemia is a macrocytic hypochromic anemia. There is a variation in the size of the red blood cells and the abnormal red blood cells do not have a normal survival time. The white blood cells are also affected in pernicious anemia (lympho-cytosis and abnormal granulocytes).

The stomach is affected by an atrophic gastritis. Gastric analysis reveals an achylia following histamine stimulation. The central nervous system changes include atrophy and degeneration of the dorsal and lateral columns of the spinal cord, degeneration of ganglion cells, and demyelination. There is also degeneration of peripheral nerves. Patients with pernicious anemia have a predisposition to carcinoma of the stomach, cirrhosis of the liver, sprue and celiac disease, pellagra, and intestinal disorders. Diarrhea, loss of weight, paresthesia, glossitis and sore tongue, and achlorhydria are the principal findings. Treatment with vitamin B_{12} produces a proliferation of normoblastic tissue which replaces the megaloblastic tissue in the bone marrow. Erythropoietic tissue is converted to normaloblastic tissue in twenty-four hours following initiation of therapy.

Aplastic anemia results from failure of blood cells to undergo maturation at an early phase. A severe anemia, leukopenia and thrombocytopenia develop. Individuals with aplastic anemia show weakness, fatigue, dyspnea, sepsis and fever, and purpuric manifestations. The anemia is common in young adult females.

Myelophthisic anemia is an anemia characterized by replacement of the bone marrow and blood-forming elements by proliferating neoplastic tissue, fibrosis of the marrow or is due to storage disease.

Diseases Due to Increased Red Blood Cells. *Polycythemia (Erythemia)* is an increase in the number of red blood cells (7 to 10 million RBC per cubic millimeter of blood). There is excessive erythroblastic activity in the bone marrow which produces a persistent polycythemia and splenomegaly.

A mild polycythemia is due to poor oxygenation. A second kind of polycythemia is of unknown etiology, i.e. polycythemia rubra. The latter occurs in middle-aged individuals and is due to a proliferation of leukopoietic (granulopoietic and erythropoietic) tissue. The red blood cells may increase to 13.5 million per cubic millimeter of blood due to overproduction rather than to increased longevity. The bone marrow is engorged and hyperplastic. Splenomegaly and hepatomegaly, ecchymoses in the skin and mucous membranes, and thrombosis are the main findings. All of the parenchymal organs are engorged and the capillaries are hyperemic. Polycythemia may be associated with a long survival period. The individual has a cyanotic appearance. Complications are due to hemorrhage and thrombosis.

ALTERATIONS IN WHITE BLOOD CELLS

Leukocytosis and Leukopenia. *Leukocytosis* is an increase in the number of circulating leukocytes. The number of immature neutrophilic leukocytes is increased in the circulating blood. Leukocytosis is present in most pyogenic infections. *Leukopenia* is a reduction in the number of circulating leukocytes. It may result from chemicals, drugs, radiation, aplasia of the bone marrow, infections, redistribution of white blood cells within the vascular channels, and increased destruction of white blood cells.

Infectious Mononucleosis. Infectious mononucleosis is an acute, benign, infectious disease of obscure etiology characterized by the following clinical findings: irregular fever, sore throat, lymphadenopathy, splenomegaly, hep-

atomegaly, purpura and jaundice. Infectious mononucleosis is characterized by a leukocytosis with atypical lymphocytes, lymphocytosis and anemia.
Infectious mononucleosis is generally self-limiting in approximately three
weeks; however, the disease has been reported to exist for weeks to as long
as months.

The clinical laboratory findings concerning infectious mononucleosis include the following: leukocytosis (10,000 to 25,000), lymphocytosis (50%
to 90%), atypical lymphocytes, normal erythrocytes, possible decreased platelets, normal bone marrow, serum heterophile agglutinin titre above 1:120
which is diagnostic, and bone marrow eosinophilia.

The lymph nodes are enlarged and show extreme hyperplasia of lymphocytes and reticulum, with atypical lymphocytes present in the sinuses.

Agranulocytosis is a marked depression in the formation of leukocytes
accompanied by a decrease in the number of granulocytes in the circulating
blood. Agranulocytosis is associated with infections, chemicals and drugs.
There is an absence of anemia.

Cyclical Neutropenia. Cyclical neutropenia is a rare periodic decrease in
circulating polymorphonuclear leukocytes. The disorder affects both males
and females and persists without remissions. The neutropenia generally follows a rhythmical pattern of three-week periodicity. Every three weeks the
following symptoms appear: anorexia, malaise, and lymphadenitis.

Leukemia. Leukemia is a neoplasm of white blood cells which terminates
fatally. Widespread proliferation of leukocytes and their precursors infiltrate the blood and tissues of the body with numerous immature and abnormal cell forms. The bone marrow is stimulated by some obscure etiologic
factor (s) into producing leukocytes or their precursors at the expense of
the normal erythroblastic tissue.

The leukemias are classified according to the type of white blood cells
produced by the leukocyte-forming tissue present in the bone marrow, i.e.
myeloid, lymphatic and monocytic. The latter three types may be acute or
chronic. Acute leukemias develop during the first decade of life; chronic
myeloid leukemia develops between twenty-five and forty-five years of age,
and chronic lymphoid leukemia develops between forty-five and sixty years
of age.

Acute leukemia develops insidiously and the neoplasm follows a rapid
course with high white blood counts, anemia and thrombocytopenia. The
bone marrow throughout the body is densely infiltrated with primitive undifferentiated white blood cells.

Chronic myeloid leukemia results from a hyperplasia of the bone marrow
with a tremendous increase in granular leukocytes in the circulating blood
and numerous immature myeloblasts and myelocytes are readily visible in
blood smears. The white blood cell count is extremely elevated and may
reach 500,000 or more per cubic millimeter. Normocytic anemia and increased platelets, and decreased erythropoiesis occurs as the bone marrow is
displaced by proliferating immature leukocytes. This leukemia follows a

chronic course and may last for one to five years terminating fatally. Chronic myeloid leukemia has the most rapid course of all chronic leukemias. The bone marrow contains predominantly myelocytes and myeloid infiltration causes an enlarged spleen and liver. Myeloid cells infiltrate the kidney, lymph nodes, heart and viscera.

Chronic lymphatic leukemia is accompanied by a white blood cell count under 100,000 lymphoid cells per cubic millimeter. Anemia results from a reduction of red blood cells. The spleen, lymph nodes and liver are infiltrated with lymphoid cells. The bone marrow is replaced by an infiltrate of mainly lymphocytes with minimal numbers of lymphoblasts. The skin contains infiltrations of lymphocytes. This leukemia has an insidious onset with weight loss, fatigue, lymphadenopathy and bone tenderness.

Monocytic leukemia occurs in the chronic form in 10 to 11 percent of instances of this leukemia. Acute monocytic leukemia is the most common form of this leukemia. Mature and immature monocytes are present in the circulating blood but in greatly increased numbers. Monocytic leukemia occurs in two types, i.e. the Naegeli type and the Schilling type. The Naegeli type consists of immature monocytes intermediate between monocytes and myeloblasts. The Schilling type consists of immature cells in the blood resembling monocytes and reticuloendothelial cells. Skin and oral mucosal infiltrations plus hyperplasia are common as well as hemorrhage from the oral and mucous membranes.

Plasma cell leukemia is more correctly termed *multiple myeloma,* i.e. abnormal plasma cells are present in the circulating blood. Multiple myeloma is a primary neoplasm of the elements of the bone marrow.

Aleukemic leukemia is characterized by splenomegaly in individuals of middle age or older. The peripheral blood may contain immature red blood cells and there is a leukocytosis with or without features of leukemia. The bone marrow may be filled with abnormal white blood cells. This reaction may represent a form of myeloid leukemia or a response of hematopoietic cells to a nonspecific stimulus and therefore may not be associated with anemia.

Diseases Associated with Elevated White Blood Cell Counts. Lymphocytosis is present in viral diseases, bacterial infections, tuberculosis, syphilis, brucellosis, infectious mononucleosis, and in convalescent patients. Elevated basophiles occur in chronic granulocytic leukemia, smallpox (variola), irradiation and polycythemia. Elevated eosinophiles are present in familial eosinophilia, allergic diseases, recovery phase of infections, parasitic infections, collagen diseases, dermatologic diseases, reticuloendotheliosis, hypoadrenal-corticism and metastatic neoplasms. Elevated neutrophiles occur in pyogenic infections, physiological neutrophilia, necrosis, neoplasms, intoxication, abnormal metabolism and polycythemia.

Diseases Associated with Lowered White Blood Cell Counts. Leukopenia is caused by irradiation, typhoid fever, chemotherapy with cytotoxic drugs, sulfonamides, thiouracil and amidopyrine. Leukopenia may be due to lymphopenia or neutropenia.

PURPURA

Thrombocytopenic Purpura. Purpura is the presence of an extravasation of blood (petechiae and ecchymosis) beneath the skin and mucous membranes of the body. Purpura accompanies various pathologic processes, i.e. leukemias, advanced anemia, and certain severe infectious diseases. *Thrombocytopenic purpura* is a specific form of purpura which is associated with a decrease in the number of blood platelets (thrombocytes) in children and young adults. The blood vessel walls undergo an alteration so that spontaneous hemorrhages occur into the mucous membranes, skin and joints. Thrombocytopenic purpura occurs secondary to systemic diseases, i.e. severe infections and septic states, meningococcus septicemia, chemicals, poisons and drugs. The disease is common in Caucasian females.

The bone marrow is normal and, therefore, platelet formation is not affected. The spleen may or may not be palpated. Females with thrombocytopenic purpura have a prolonged and heavy menstruation. Small hemorrhages occur in the central nervous system. In rare instances, platelet agglutination occurs. The latter patients are destroying their own platelets. The cause of platelet agglutination is unknown.

Thrombotic Thrombocytopenic Purpura. This rare condition is a disease of the arterioles and capillaries characterized by platelet thromboses, hemolytic anemia, thrombocytopenic purpura, fever and neurological disturbances. The arterioles and capillaries are occluded by hyaline or eosinophilic (fibrinoid) material. The spleen is congested and enlarged and there is a reduction in blood platelets to less than 50,000 per cubic millimeter. This purpura is fatal in a matter of weeks. The etiology is currently obscure; however, the disease has similarities to the collagen diseases.

HEMOPHILIAS

Hemophilia is an inherited disease transmitted as a recessive sex-linked Mendelian factor. Females carry the gene, but the disease appears only in males.

Classic hemophilia "A" is due to deficiency of antihemophilic globulin (AHG). Blood coagulation is prolonged; however, the following hematologic tests are normal: bleeding time, clot retraction, prothrombin concentration, and the tourniquet test. The platelets fail to release thromboplastin. Prolonged hemorrhage results from trauma. Hemarthroses produces painful and deformed joints.

Christmas disease or hemophilia "B" is due to a deficiency of plasma thromboplastic component (PTC). The deficiency is a sex-linked Mendelian recessive disease. The findings are petechiae and ecchymoses in the mucous membrane and skin, epistaxis, and hemarthrosis which are all of a lesser severity than the manifestations of hemophilia "A."

Hemophilia "C" is due to a rare deficiency of plasma thromboplastic antecedent (PTA) or factor XI. The disease affects both males and females. The genetic nature of this disease is obscure; however, it is not a sex-linked Mendelian recessive disease. The clinical manifestations of hemophilia C are milder than those of hemophilia A.

Von Willebrand's disease is a hereditary hematologic disorder of obscure etiology which affects both males and females. The platelet count is normal, the bleeding time is prolonged, the clotting time and clot retraction are normal; however, there is increased capillary fragility. Females with this disorder bleed heavily during menstruation.

Chapter 18

DISEASES OF THE SKELETAL SYSTEM

INFECTIONS OF BONE

Acute Osteomyelitis. Osteomyelitis of bone and bones is produced by various pyogenic microorganisms. The most common organisms provoking osteomyelitis are *Staphylococcus aureus,* beta-hemolytic streptococcus and pneumococcus. The latter microorganisms reach bone tissue by the following means: through a fracture, spreading from adjacent tissues, or by way of the blood stream from a distant inflammation. The microorganisms may be cultured from the blood of infected subjects. When the site of inflammation is localized to the periosteum the infection is termed periostitis. When the site of inflammation is present in bone tissue the term *osteitis* is used. During osteomyelitis, the periosteum, bone marrow, and bone tissue are all involved. Acute osteomyelitis occurs in childhood and is rare in adults. Suppuration develops in the medullary cavity of the long bones and spreads widely accompanied by bone pain, fever and leukocytosis. Radiographic examination of the infected bones during the early stage of osteomyelitis fails to reveal any significant alterations in bone tissue. The suppuration may burrow through a thin cortex in the metaphysis (shaft of long bone) to reach the periosteum. The periosteum is not attached very strongly to the shaft of the infected long bone. The infection spreads to form a subperiosteal abscess which encompasses a large area of the shaft in pus.

The epiphysial plate (cartilage) is a barrier to the spread of osteomyelitis from the metaphysis (extremity of shaft) to the epiphysis (extremity). Areas of bone tissue adjacent to the pus and colonies of microorganisms become necrotic and the dead bone is separated from the living bone to form a sequestrum. In severe instances the entire diaphysis (shaft) may become necrotic and become separated from the epiphysis in the form of a large sequestrum. The portion of a sequestrum covered by pus remains unaltered; however, resorption of bone may take place if granulation tissue is present adjacent to an area of the sequestrum. When the acute osteomyelitis passes into the subacute phase, new bone is deposited beneath the periosteum to shield the dead bone. The newly deposited bone is termed an *involucrum.* The involucrum contains perforations termed *cloaca* through which the pus drains. The presence of a sequestrum is responsible for the continuation of the infection and retardation of the healing process. The sequestrum which is surrounded by pus cannot undergo dissolution and resolution. A chronic

deposit bone apatite. The osteoblasts, however, undergo normal proliferation and osteoid tissue is normally produced.

Osteomalacia, if mild, results in occasional bone pain. There is failure or delayed healing of fractures. The callus of the healing fracture is formed of osteoid tissue in place of calcified bone tissue. Severe osteomalacia is accompanied by weakening and softening of bones and radiographically decreased density of bone tissue. The most prominent alterations occur in bones with the greatest rate of bone remodeling, i.e. in cancellous bone. Microscopically, the bones with osteomalacia show osteoid tissue encompassing mineralized bone trabeculae.

Hypervitaminosis D. Excessive administration of vitamin D causes increased blood calcium and an increase of calcium and phosphorus in the urine. Widespread metastatic calcification and renal calculi may develop. Where calcium is not consumed in the diet, the increased blood calcium is the result of diminishing calcium in the bone tissue and the addition of calcium to the blood.

SKELETAL LESIONS IN ENDOCRINE DISORDERS

Primary Hyperparathyroidism. Excessive parathyroid hormone acts directly on bone tissue. Primary hyperparathyroidism causes increased resorption of bone tissue. Osteoclasts and Howship's lacunae are abundant on the surface of bone trabeculae. Osteoblasts are also prominent; therefore, resorption and apposition of bone are both active processes during hyperparathyroidism. The bone marrow is subsequently replaced by fibrous connective tissue and the disease is termed *osteitis fibrosa*. New formation of bone trabeculae occurs in loose fibrous vascular tissue. A large number of giant cells are present in the connective tissue forming the brown tumor or giant cell tumor of hyperparathyroidism. When the parathyroid tumor is excised from the neck, the serum calcium drops, osteoclastic activity becomes normal, and the bone tissue becomes normal.

Secondary Hyperparathyroidism. Chronic renal failure, associated with a decrease in serum calcium, may produce alterations in bone tissue. The bone changes are identical to those seen in primary hyperparathyroidism.

Acromegaly. Enlarged mandible and enlarged hands and feet are due to acromegaly. During acromegaly, there is subperiosteal proliferation and endochondral ossification in specific bones (ribs, vertebrae and digits) of the skeleton. The overgrowth of bone tissue is readily discernible in the skull, face and mandible, and extremities. Acromegaly is due to an adenoma of the pituitary gland which develops after completion of bone growth.

Cushing's Syndrome. This syndrome is accompanied by osteoporosis. The vertebrae contain decreased or an absence of the cortical plate and the individual bone trabeculae are small and thin. This syndrome is primarily an adrenal cortical disturbance; however, identical skeletal alterations result following excessive dosages of cortisone therapy. Prolonged cortisone therapy produces alterations in the basophils of the pituitary gland.

Cretinism. Cretinism produces retardation of endochrondal growth due to hypoplasia or lack of development of the thyroid gland. The epiphyses of the long bones are deformed and may be delayed in their closure. Ossification is also delayed in cretinism.

Hyperthyroidism. A hyperplastic and overactive thyroid is associated with a mild osteoporosis of the skeleton. Bone resorption occurs at a greater rate than bone apposition. The bony alterations in hyperthyroidism are dependent upon the grade of the severity of the disease since nodular goiters produce less severe manifestations than diffuse thyroid, and hypertrophy and hyperplasia of the thyroid gland.

TABLE XXIV

SYNDROMES OF THE PARATHYROID GLAND

Primary Hyperparathyroidism
>   Etiology—Adenoma, primary hyperplasia, primary carcinoma
>   (rarely) of parathyroid glands
>   Elevated serum calcium (hypercalcemia)
>   Decreased serum phosphorus
>   Elevated serum alkaline phosphatase
>   Elevated urinary calcium
>   Elevated urinary phosphorus
>   Normal stool calcium
>   Normal stool phosphorus
>   Demineralization of bone tissue
>   Increased resorption of bone tissue, active formation of osteoid tissue
>   Bone pain, pathologic fractures, shortened skeleton
>   Radiolucent lesions in long bones, vertebrae, skull and jaws
>   Local decalcification, cysts, giant cell tumors (Brown tumors)
>   Generalized skeletal disease is termed osteitis fibrosa cystics (von
>   Recklinghausen's disease of bone)
>   Abdominal Pain, peptic ulcers, constipation due to hypercalcemia
>   Nephrolithiasis (renal stones or calculi) and urinary calculi
>   Nephrocalcinosis (metastatic calcification in renal tubules)
>   Metastatic calcification in muscular arteries
>   Renal and skeletal alterations preventable
>   Clinical chemistry is less reliable following development of renal
>   failure

Secondary Hyperparathyroidism
>   Associated with chronic renal disease (renal insufficiency, phosphate
>   retention and stimulation of parathyroid)
>   All parathyroid glands are enlarged—no neoplasia present
>   Renal failure and metabolic acidosis
>   Decreased serum calcium
>   Elevated serum alkaline phosphatase
>   Decreased urinary calcium
>   Decreased urinary phosphorus
>   Generalized skeletal disease (osteitis fibrosa cystica or von
>   Recklinghausen's disease of bone)
>   Increased resorption of bone tissue
>   Demineralization of bone tissue
>   Renal and skeletal alterations not preventable

Hypoparathyroidism
>   Etiology—removal of parathyroid glands during surgery in neck
>   region
>   Lack of bone resorption (decreased osteoclasts)
>   Bone tissue thicker than normal
>   Hyposecretion of parathyroid hormone
>   Decreased serum calcium
>   Elevated serum phosphorus
>   Decreased serum alkaline phosphatase
>   Decreased urinary phosphorus
>   Decreased urinary calcium
>   Tetany
>   Minimal to no organ alterations

BONE DISORDERS OF OBSCURE ETIOLOGY

Osteoporosis. Osteoporosis is a decrease in the quantity of calcified bone tissue in a given amount of skeletal tissue. The matrix of skeletal tissue appears to be normally mineralized. This disorder may be due to either decreased bone apposition or increased bone resorption, or a combination of these conditions. The etiology is obscure. However, there is an increase in the incidence of fractures, deformities and altered bone and bones. The following forms of osteoporosis may develop: localized, generalized, disuse atrophy and immobilization osteoporosis, and senile osteoporosis. Hormonal alterations such as insufficient or absence of estrogen appears to produce osteoporosis. However, the etiology of osteoporosis is obscure. Histopathologically, the bones show thin trabeculae and a decrease in cortical bone. The following diseases are associated with generalized osteoporosis: Cushing's syndrome, acromegaly, and thyrotoxicosis.

Paget's Disease of Bone. Paget's disease of bone is a chronic osteodystrophy of bone tissue of unknown etiology which occurs after forty or fifty years of age. Males are affected more than females. The alkaline phosphatase level of the blood is increased, otherwise the blood biochemistry is normal. This unusual bone disease is characterized by increased osteoblastic activity simultaneous with osteoclastic resorption of bone. The overgrowth of new bone tissue consists of a poorly calcified bone containing rather irregular spicules of bone. An individual bone may be affected in a small percentage of instances; however, the vertebrae, cranium, sternum, femur, tibia, sacrum, pelvis and jaws are commonly involved. The condition is not considered a diffuse disease of bone tissue, rather it is a multifocal bone disease. Advanced instances of Paget's disease are accompanied by tenderness and bone pain, bowing of the lower extremities, and an increase in skull size and an increase in jaw size. Osteogenic sarcoma may develop in three percent of advanced or terminal instances of this bone disease.

The bones of the skeleton become thickened but are soft, porous and therefore light in weight. The skull shows a severe thickening of the calvarium which is a progressive change. Microscopically, simultaneous apposition and irregular resorption of bone are present. The marrow becomes fibrotic and the vascularity of the bone marrow is increased. Early microscopic findings of Paget's disease reveal activity of both the osteoclasts and osteoblasts. Initially, the bone resorption is marked and the bone lighter than normal. The latter bone is subject to bowing and/or fracture. As the disease progresses, the bone trabeculae are commonly thickened with the development of the mosaic pattern. The pathognomonic and diagnostic mosaic pattern consists of numerous irregular cement lines which result following repeated resorption and apposition of bone. In the advanced stages the bone becomes heavier but weaker than normal. The weakened bone makes it susceptible to fracture. Osteoarthritis may follow bone deformities resulting in abnormal stresses on the major joints.

Fibrous Dysplasia. Monostotic and polyostotic fibrous dysplasia are benign fibro-osseous lesions of bone of obscure etiology. On rare occasions the polyostotic form of fibrous dysplasia of bone is associated with pigmentation of the skin, precocious sexual maturation in girls, and precocious skeletal development. The latter symptom complex is termed *Albright's syndrome.* Monostotic fibrous dysplasia generally occurs in a rib, mandible, maxilla, skull, femur and tibia. Polyostotic fibrous dysplasia frequently occurs in the femur and tibia, although many bones may be affected.

The lesions of fibrous dysplasia are accompanied by a thin cortex. The bone marrow and trabeculae are replaced by a white firm fibro-osseous tissue with a gritty consistency. Focal cystic degeneration and areas of cartilage may be present in lesions of fibrous dysplasia. Radiographically, the area of fibrous dysplasia has a ground-glass appearance with fine mottling due to the presence of woven bone. Fibrous dysplasia of the skull and jaws generally tends to contain more dense bone tissue than lesions in other sites. Therefore, upon radiographic examination, they appear more mottled and may contain areas of sclerosis.

Microscopically, the marrow and spongiosa are replaced by loose fibrous connective tissue with spindle-shaped cells. In the latter stroma are small, curved and irregular trabeculae of poorly calcified, nonlamellar woven bone tissue. The bone trabeculae are irregularly scattered throughout the fibrous stroma. Osteoblasts are not present along the borders of individual bone trabeculae. The newly deposited trabeculae fail to undergo maturation to mature lamellar bone tissue. Pain and bone deformity begins during childhood and adolescent years with the fibrous dysplasia following a slowly progressive course.

DEVELOPMENTAL ABNORMALITIES OF BONE TISSUE

Osteopetrosis. Marble bone disease or Albers-Schönberg disease (osteopetrosis) is a hereditary, Mendelian recessive disorder of bone tissue characterized by a great increase in the thickness and excessive density of all bones. The bone marrow is obliterated and a severe osteosclerotic anemia develops. In spite of the increased thickness and excessive density of the bones, fractures and brittle, chalky bones are present. The base of the skull, femur, tibia, pelvis, and vertebrae are the most commonly affected bones. Complications include deafness and impaired vision following involvement of the skull.

Osteogenesis Imperfecta. Osteogenesis imperfecta is a familial and hereditary condition which develops during intrauterine life. A mesenchymal hypoplasia with marked alterations in the bones is present at birth. The mesenchymal hypoplasia produces fragile bone with repeated spontaneous fractures. As a result of numerous irregular fractures the bones are shortened and have an altered morphology. In osteogenesis imperfecta fractures and callus formation may occur before birth. The cranium is softened and there is deficient ossification of cranial bones. The bones have a thin cortex and decreased quantity of cancellous tissues. Bone trabeculae are sparse and thin. Healing (callus) occurs following the numerous fractures; however, the bone is poorly ossified. The proliferation of cartilage cells (chondrocytes) in the epiphyseal plate is unaltered and ossification of cartilage matrix in the zone of ossification proceeds in a normal fashion. However, there is a decreased quantity of bone formed. Deafness due to otosclerosis may develop in adults with osteogenesis imperfecta.

Achondroplasia. This developmental abnormality of bone is a frequent form of dwarfism resulting from the failure of endochondral ossification. Dwarfism is present at birth and the characteristic features include the following: head appears large, extremely short but thick bones in all extremities, nose is sunken, and skin of the extremities is folded. The bones of the head and trunk develop to a normal size. The soft tissues undergo excessive growth. The short thick bone in the extremities results from deficient endochondral growth and ossification.

PRIMARY NEOPLASMS OF BONE TISSUE

Primary neoplasms of bone tissue are of mesenchymal origin. The latter neoplasms arise from fibrous tissue (fibroma and fibrosarcoma), cartilage (enchondroma and chondrosarcoma), bone (osteoma, osteoid osteoma, benign osteoblastoma, osteosarcoma and parosteal osteosarcoma), unknown origin (giant cell tumor-benign and malignant), vascular tissue (hemangioma, glomus tumor and hemangio-endothelioma), fat cells (lipoma and liposarcoma) marrow elements (solitary plasmacytoma and myelomatosis), marrow stroma (reticulum cell sarcoma) and neural tissue (schwannoma, neurofibromatosis, ganglioneuroma and neurofibrosarcoma).

Certain benign neoplasms of bone may progress to malignancy. This group includes the osteocartilaginous exostosis, enchondroma, giant cell tumor, solitary plasmacytoma and neurofibromatosis.

The osteoma occurs as a bony prominence on bones of the skull and jaws and may protrude into the orbit, paranasal sinuses and oral cavity. The osteoma is benign and consists of connective tissue and spongy bone trabeculae or of very dense compact bone.

The osteogenic sarcoma is a malignant neoplasm of bone arising from the undifferentiated bone-forming mesenchyme. This sarcoma is the most common primary malignant neoplasm of bone tissue. It occurs more often in males than females from ten to twenty-five years of age. The most common site is in the metaphysis of long bones, around the knee, and upper end of the femur and humerus. The neoplasm produces severe pain and swelling, but the patient is in good health provided no metastases have taken place. Spread of the osteogenic sarcoma occurs by way of the blood stream to the lungs, viscera, and other bones. The prognosis is poor with a five year survival rate of from 5 to 20 percent.

Osteocartilaginous exostosis is a very common benign neoplasm or bony mass. It is comprised of an inner core of cancellous bone covered by cartilage

TABLE XXV

DIFFERENTIATING FEATURES OF GIANT CELL TUMOR, BONE CYST AND
OSTEOGENIC SARCOMA

Giant Cell Tumor	*Bone Cyst*	*Osteogenic Sarcoma*
Asymmetrical bone destruction in epiphysis extending to joint cartilage	Occurrence in childhood Pathologic fracture without preceding symptoms	Central destruction in shaft of long bone with symmetrical expansion of bone shell
Occurrence in adult		Sclerosis of cancellous bone with new bone formation in metaphysis
Bone destruction, pain and swelling in lower end of radius, upper end of tibia or lower femur		Occurs in adolescence or post adolescence
		Periosteal lipping
		Groomed whiskers in radiograph

and perichondrium. The exostosis may be single or multiple and arise predominantly from the metaphyses of the femur, humerus and tibia.

The enchondroma is a benign cartilagenous neoplasm arising within the medullary cavity of small bones of the hands and feet. The cartilagenous growth may be single or multiple and appears radiolucent. Symptoms include pain unassociated with fracture, enlargement of long bones, swelling and pathological fracture in the phalangeal lesions.

Chondrosarcoma is a malignant neoplasm of bone which either begins as a primary growth or starts as a benign cartilagenous neoplasm which undergoes malignant transformation. This neoplasm occurs within and on the surface of bones. It occurs in males twice as often as in females from forty to seventy years of age. The neoplasm arises in the ribs, pelvis and the proximal femur. Chondrosarcoma has been difficult to diagnosis and biopsies should be taken from the proliferating edge and not from the calcified or degenerated cartilage. The chondrosarcoma has a chronic or prolonged course with metastases developing by way of the blood stream to the lungs and the neoplasm spreads along veins in a retrograde fashion. Prognosis is poor to guarded because of misdiagnosis by pathologists.

The fibrosarcoma is a rare malignant tumor of bone. It occurs both within and on the surface of bones in adults. It affects the metaphysis of long bones around the knee joint. The endosteal fibrosarcoma occurs within the medullary cavity of bones and has a poor prognosis. The peripheral fibrosarcoma on the surface of bones has a prognosis which is directly related to the degree of cell differentiation. Highly collageneous peripheral fibrosarcomas metastasize late and have a good prognosis. Undifferentiated pleomorphic peripheral fibrosarcomas metastasize early and have a poor prognosis.

Giant-cell tumors of bone produce an osteolytic lesion in the end of a long bone of individuals from twenty to forty years of age. Fifty percent of the giant-cell tumors develop around the knee, i.e. in the lower end of the femur or upper end of the tibia. Approximately 50 percent of the giant-cell tumors are treated successfully by local excision. However, one-third recur and 15 to 20 percent are malignant either initially or following recurrence and metastasize to the lungs. Some giant-cell tumors which appear microscopically benign have been known to metastasize later.

the tendon sheath (villo-nodular synovitis) and the synovial sarcoma. The

rare synovial sarcoma is highly malignant and occurs outside a joint in young adults. Metastases are common to the lungs, lymph nodes and parenchymal organs. Prognosis is bad and the mortality rate is high.

Voluntary Muscle. Traumatic myositis ossificans is a benign lesion of voluntary muscle resulting from a single or multiple injury. There is proliferation of fibrous connective tissue within the affected muscle and metaplastic bone tissue is laid down in this fibroblastic proliferation. Bone may form directly in the connective tissue or cartilage may be laid down and later undergo ossification. Bacterial myositis of voluntary muscle results following gas gangrene, suppuration, Zenker's degeneration, and viral and parasitic myositis.

TABLE XXIX
CHARACTERISTICS OF SPECIFIC FORMS OF ARTHRITIS

Characteristic	Form of Arthritis
Tophi	Gout (Panarthritis)
Osteophytes	Osteoarthritis (traumatic)
Rheumatoid nodule	Rheumatoid arthritis
Rice bodies	Tuberculous arthritis
Big, boggy, broken down, painless joint	Syphilitic arthritis
Heberden's node	Osteoarthritis
Pannus	Rheumatoid arthritis
Gibbus	Tuberculous arthritis
Podagra	Gout
Pain and swelling with return to normal	Palindromic arthritis

TABLE XXX
DIFFERENTIATING FEATURES OF RHEUMATOID ARTHRITIS, OSTEOARTHRITIS AND GOUT

Rheumatoid Arthritis	Osteoarthritis	Gout
Pain increasing on work and activity	Stiffness disappearing as day wears on	Onset of acute pain and swelling in sleep
Elevation blood sedimentation rate	Occurring postmenopausally in obese women often with hypertension	Elevated serum uric acid
Onset in young adults with symmetrical joints involved		Occurrence predominantly in males in certain families
	Central erosion of joint cartilage	Punched out areas in ends of small bones

TABLE XXXI
TYPES OF DERMATITIS AND COLLAGEN DISEASES ASSOCIATED WITH RHEUMATOID ARTHRITIS

Disseminated Lupus Erythematosus
Psoriasis
Periarteritis
Rheumatic fever

TABLE XXXII
DISEASES GIVING RISE TO JOINT MICE

Osteoarthritis—fractured meniscus
Tuberculosis—Rice bodies
Osteochondromatosis
Osteochondritis dissecans

TABLE XXXIII

DISEASES PRODUCING AN ELEVATION OF SERUM ALKALINE PHOSPHATASE	DISEASES PRODUCING DECREASED SERUM ALKALINE PHOSPHATASE
Primary hyperparathyroidism	Cretinism (Congenital Hypo- thyroidism at Birth)
Secondary hyperparathyroidism (renal rickets)	Jaundice (Icterus)
Multiple myeloma	Scurvy
Osteomalacia	Achondroplasia
Paget's disease	Congenital Hypophosphatasia
Rachitic tetany	
Rickets	
Caffey's disease (infantile cortical hyperostosis)	
Osteosarcoma	
Sarcoidosis	
Albright's syndrome	
Alber's-Schonberg disease (osteopetrosis)	
Biliary obstruction	
Liver abscess	
Portal cirrhosis	
Hyperthyroidism	
Pregnancy	
Gestation	

APPENDIX

NORMAL VALUES

RBC female	4,800,000 cells/cu mm
RBC male	5,400,000 cells/cu mm
RBC children	5,040,000 cells/cu mm
Hemoglobin (Male)	13–20 gm/100 ml
Hemoglobin (Female)	11–18 gm/100 ml
Blood Glucose	70–100 mg/100 ml of whole blood
Non Protein Nitrogen (NPN)	25–35 mg/100 ml
Total Cholesterol	150–270 mg/100 ml
Serum Alkaline Phosphatase	2–4 Bodansky units or 3–13 King-Armstrong units per 100 ml
Serum Inorganic Phosphorus	3–5 mg/100 ml
Serum calcium	9–11 mg/100 ml
Sedimentation Rate	Males, 3.7 mm/hr Females, 9.6 mm/hr
Serum Protein	6.5–8.2% (gm/100 cc) albumin 4.6% (gm/100 ml) globulin 1.2% (gm/100 ml)
Clotting time (coagulation time)	5 to 15 minutes
Bleeding time	1 to 3 or 8 minutes, may be prolonged to 8 minutes.
Protein Bound Iodine (PBI)	4 to 6 gamma per 100 ml of blood
Creatinine	1–2 mg/100 ml of whole blood
Icteric index (serum)	4 to 6
Segmented smears (Differential leukocyte count)	
Neutrophiles	60–70%
Lymphocytes	20–30%
Monocytes	2–6%
Eosinophiles	1–4%
Basophiles	0.5%
WBC	7,000 per cu mm
Platelets	150,000 to 400,000 per cu mm

INDEX

185